Three Forms of
Sudden Death

Three Forms of Sudden Death

AND OTHER REFLECTIONS ON THE GRANDEUR AND MISERY OF THE BODY

F. Gonzalez-Crussi

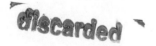

1817

HARPER & ROW, PUBLISHERS, NEW YORK

Cambridge, Philadelphia, San Francisco, Washington
London, Mexico City, São Paulo, Singapore, Sydney

Portions of this work originally appeared in somewhat different form in *The Sciences.*

FIRST EDITION

Designer: Helene Berinsky

Library of Congress Cataloging-in-Publication Data

Gonzalez-Crussi, F.
    Three forms of sudden death.

    1. Body, Human. 2. Human physiology—Popular works.
3. Sudden death. 4. Human growth. I. Title.
QP38.G66   1986   612   86-45108
ISBN 0-06-015629-5

86 87 88 89 90 RRD 10 9 8 7 6 5 4 3 2 1

To my mother, María de Jesús

Contents

Three Forms of
Sudden Death

Generation: Past, Present, and Future

Generation, that portentous biologic phenomenon, did not seem to the ancients especially difficult to understand. Aristotle gave them a very convenient handle by which to grasp an otherwise bewildering natural occurrence when he said: "The reality of things resides in form; matter is mere potentiality." The statue of Hermes, by way of example, acquires reality the moment the hands of the sculptor confer form to the raw marble or the uncarved wood; form is what is added: the form conceived in the mind of the artist, and nothing else. Likewise, the sage lives as potentiality in the uneducated man, but may receive form if the latter is susceptible to learning. Clearly, the Aristotelian "form"—*morphé*—is something much more complex than the simple "shape" of an object. It is that which gives unity to individual things, their very essence. Thus, the Stagirite's system soon confronts us with a series of abstract statements: Form is superior to matter, because it is more "actual." The soul is the form of the body. And it is the soul that perceives, since the body, being pure matter, is unsentient. God is all Form and pure "actuality," therefore unchangeable. In contrast, living beings are a combination of form and matter. But since matter is neither created nor destroyed, when a living being is created it is solely the form that has a beginning. Matter is never in short supply. Therefore, all that is required to bring about the emergence of form is just a tiny spark, as it were, of energy. And when it comes to human generation, matter is supplied by women, and form, by men.

Matter is furnished by Woman, of course. It could not be otherwise, for the maternal element represents the passive earth, and earth is one of the four elements (only four!) that enter into the composition of all matter in the universe. Motion, activity, energy, reside in the masculine—the manly is identified with the sun in all ancient religions—and energy alone can confer form. The belief thus emerged that women carry in the womb all matter necessary for procreation, but the energy necessary for activating this matter and giving it form is contained in the male seed only. This belief solidified into the rocklike immutability that is proper to Aristotelian doctrine. Eighteen centuries later, Montaigne was to write that just as land that lies fallow will sprout all sorts of wild and useless weeds, but can be turned into a garden plot when sown with the right seed, "so women by themselves succeed in producing only heaps and pieces of formless flesh, but must be burthen'd with another [male] seed to produce a wholesome and natural offspring" (Book 1, chap. 8).

Spontaneous generation, in this system, is hardly an absurdity. It is, rather, a logical necessity. For all that is required to create a new living being is to effect a few minor rearrangements in the four elements that compose matter. At most, a few permutations here and there. No wonder, then, that when the sun rays pierce through the foliage in the woods and fall upon the mud at the foot of an umbrous tree, worms and tadpoles, and insects and snakes spring forth! Indeed, everyone can verify that when these light beams enter the crevices of a felled tree trunk, or a decomposing carcass in the forest, insects swarm by the thousands, bees fly about, and countless grubs writhe out of the decaying mass. Varro (116–27 B.C.), like most of his contemporaries, believed that bees could be descended from bees, or from rotting carcasses of oxen, "which is why Archelaus calls

them 'winged offspring of the putrescent ox' in an epigram."
And up to the seventeenth century, when Aristotelianism was
openly challenged, it was admitted that complex animals like
mice could originate spontaneously from an appropriate material substratum. Jean Baptiste Van Helmont (1577–1644), Bel-
gian physician and harsh critic of Aristotle (on the grounds that
no pagan should be admitted as contributor to a scientific
edifice that must be based wholly on Christian thought), left us
a recipe for generating a mouse. This protocol, whose precise
demands render it worthy of the name "experimental," goes
something like this: Place in a container a few rags, and bran,
and leave it in a corner of your attic. Under carefully controlled
conditions of temperature and humidity, it is guaranteed that
after two or three days at least one mouse will have formed.

However, man's origins could not be put on a par with the
procreation of these base creatures. Other hypotheses had to be
constructed that reckoned with our superiority; and one can
always count on our abysmal self-complacency to support theories that glorify our condition. Vanity entered greatly in the
early taxonomy that segregated living beings into two classes
according to their mode of generation. One large class com-
prises "all that is born of putrid and muddy matter," and another class, where man belongs, includes the most perfect beings, those born by insemination. The gestation of the former
is random, instantaneous, and indiscriminate as to site; that of
the latter must take place inside the maternal womb, amidst the
warmth, silence, and unperturbed stillness that alone can ensure the ripening of the richest fruits, or the crystallization of
the rarest pearls. But this arrogance of the early naturalists, who
placed man highest in the hierarchy of the biologic scale, was
countered by the Church with this humbling reminder: all that
is corruptible is made of matter, and matter is close to nothingness, since it was barely drawn out of nothingness by the Creator. Accordingly, Saint Anselm and Saint Bonaventure extend
the hierarchical system of creatures in an upward direction.
Above the beings created by insemination, there are semi-cor-

poreal beings of incorruptible nature generated by divine fiat: these are called angels. And above these, there are still higher beings: archangels. And above these, yet higher beings, closer to the glory of the Creator, called cherubs. And so on. So that contemplation of the created universe cannot fill the observer with the sin of pride. However refined or mysterious man's gestation may be, however hidden and exalted a process, it is still an imprinting of form upon matter. And the precarious existence of matter proves that it is next to nothingness, always close to return to the nothingness whence it came. It is a healthy duty to remember that, in the extended scale of created beings, man's position remains a lowly one.

With the passing of centuries, the teaching of this lesson in humility devolved upon the naturalists. Lazzaro Spallanzani (1729–99) demonstrated that mice, frogs, and other creatures formerly believed to arise from miry dregs and foul residues are, like man, generated by insemination. Nor was insemination necessarily achieved inside the maternal womb. Spallanzani showed that frogs' eggs in fresh water produce tadpoles, but fail to do so in the absence of the male's seminal fluid. In conflict with the teachings of the Church (he, who eventually took orders in the Church), he carried on experiments in artificial insemination. Using techniques that he himself developed, he was able to artificially inseminate a bitch that, sixty-two days after the experiment, was delivered of three healthy puppies. To conduct his researches he contrived to design bathing trunks for male frogs: once clad in these "chastity belts," they would become incapable of procreating. One cannot fail to wonder how the agencies that support biomedical research today would react to the proposal of an investigator that showed this kind of sartorial inventiveness. And yet, all this clever experimental design allowed only limited conclusions. Granted that the seminal fluid is required for procreation, in man as well as in frog; granted that this fluid needs to be delivered into the female genital tract, in man as well as in mouse; what is the nature of this seed that is deposited, and in what way does it act?

In principle, the male seed did not have to be made up exclusively of formed matter. It could be, for aught we know, a sort of vapor ascending into the womb, a kind of airy factor rising from the seminal fluid to activate the development of a new living being in some kind of material substratum furnished by the mother. Aristotle had spoken of it as "heat," and never one to leave threadbare concepts, he supplied all sorts of corollaries: boys were more likely to be produced if copulation took place when invigorating winds were blowing; girls would be engendered if copulation was practiced when cool southern breezes were blowing; cold water could cause infertility; and the like. The idea that the male seed's active principle was "heat" gave Van Helmont the opportunity for this sarcastic retort: fish are cold-blooded, yet they may be numbered among the most prolific of living beings. But all the sarcasm distilled by Aristotle's foes could not expunge the feeling that something mysterious, unfathomable, elusive, must reside in the male's ejaculate. Zeno taught that the sperm discharged by man contains an essence mixed in the fluid, which partakes of the qualities of the man's spirit, passed on to him by his forebears; for only thus could one explain its formative powers, and its mysterious ability to reproduce in the offspring (after being absorbed by a similar female essence) the features and propensities of the begetter. A belief that holds sway for more than twenty centuries cannot be called, without injustice, sheer superstition. There were, after all, some empirical observations that favored the insubstantial nature of the inseminating male's fluid. For one thing, the male's ejaculate is not retained inside the female's body; nevertheless insemination is achieved. And then, there were numerous reports of women who conceived despite lack of penetration by the male. (Concerning the latter data, one cannot help wondering whether this was the beginning of the time-honored propensity to exaggerate observations.) Perhaps the tendency to regard man's power of procreation as an ethereal attribute lives in our subconscious. A recently retired physician once told me that, in his student days, the supervisor of a nurses' school (herself a registered nurse, and thus reasonably well versed in biology) never allowed her students into the same swimming pool where male medical students had splashed about hours before. This rule stemmed from the prudent surmise that male ejaculates could be present in the water that might have—just might have—retained their inseminating potency, thus risking the accidental impregnation of the girls entrusted to her care!

And yet, the discovery of the material nature of sperm came with such trumpeting and flourish as rarely attends the quiet toils of biologic research. It was achieved not by a learned professor but by an unschooled clerk in a dry-goods store who had taken up lens grinding as a hobby. He was constrained to report his findings to the Royal Society of London in awkward letters couched in conversational Dutch, unable to communicate in the scientific language of his day, Latin. Anthony Leeuwenhoek had, in effect, opened the astonished eyes of the world to the unperceived beauty and structural intricacy of the common objects of nature; leaves, whalebones, scales of fish, heads of flies, hairs offered unsuspected, exquisite details of morphologic organization when seen through his magnifying lenses. He had shaken the scientific world of his time with the mind-boggling discovery that infinitesimally small living beings, as numerous as the inhabitants of his hometown of Delft, in Holland, could be seen gyrating and dancing inside a single drop of water. Simple, common water, collected from the eaves of a rooftop, or from one of the low canals of the town. All this he had done, by the time he placed a few drops of viscous seminal fluid—but this pious, staunch Protestant insisted in telling us that it was not his own—under his bits of glass. And the spectacle of myriad "worms" darting in all directions, swimming indefatigably, propelled by undulating movements of their long tails, evokes in him the most intoxicating rapture, a fascination that cannot be described. But when the general stupefaction subsides, one thing is clear: Aristotle was wrong, after all. The male seed is not abstract "form," it is concrete matter, and living matter at that. And quite apart from the scientific merits of Leeuwenhoek's

discovery, the scientific community readily embraced it because it accorded with prevailing notions of male superiority.
For it became apparent that the generational faculty is essen-
tially a male prerogative. In keeping with the elevated dignity
that nature everywhere grants to the male of the species, the
precious germ out of which a human being develops is produced by the male, and by the male only. Woman is mere
receptacle and nourishment. She is the soil that receives, nur-
tures, and shelters the living seed.

But it was not enough to demonstrate that self-propelling
"animalcules," or "worms," consistently populate the seminal
fluid. It was still necessary to prove that they are fundamentally
linked with procreation. In effect, what possible relationship
could there be between these tireless microscopic beings that
undulate "like a snake held by its two extremes," and a ruddy,
wholesome newborn human infant? To many illustrious minds,
none whatsoever. Spallanzani maintained, to his death, that
spermatozoa were simple "parasites," or as we would say today,
"contaminants," without any role in the generative process.
With discursive Gallic flair, Pierre Dionis had written in his
Dissertation sur la génération de l'homme (Paris, 1698) that it
was impossible to imagine that a single spermatozoon could
fertilize the egg, for it was absurd that nature would produce
millions of sperm cells each time, when only one was necessary.
Alas, since then we have learned that all the *bon sens* in the
world counts for little when nature wishes to be extravagant,
and that her random prodigality shows little concern for our
individuality. For our precious existence comes about as in a
lottery: through the chancy biologic success of one sperm cell
—one among millions of others like it, any one of which could
have fertilized the egg. It may shock our sense of self-esteem,
but our coming into being has less the appearance of a purposeful design by a loving Providence concerned with us as individuals, and more the looks of an accident. We would not be
ourselves if a different sperm cell had succeeded. Each sperm
cell carries genes in different arrangement, and although some

similarities are to be expected in sperm cells from the same progenitor, no two cells are identical. The differences between siblings (which may include different sex) show that the individual makeup determined by different sperm cells may be astonishingly diverse. Thus, as surely as we are here today, we might have never been—save for an accident. But in a world like ours, accidents will happen. The religious viewpoint has generally been averse to this interpretation, but, it seems, not uniformly so. Salvador E. Luria, Nobel Prize-laureate physiologist, recounts a custom of certain groups of orthodox Jews that seems to have taken into consideration the randomness of our origin.[1] In funeral processions, the sons were forbidden to follow their father's bier. And this prohibition seems to have been based on the belief that the flesh-and-blood descendants should have some regard for the uncreated progeny, "the beings that might have been but never were." In other words, the unrealized offspring in the spilled or wasted seed of the father were assumed to remain capable of attending the funeral. Moreover, their immaterial status did not preclude their feeling envy, and the prohibition imposed on the "real" sons was designed to safeguard them from the potential rancor that the "unreal" descendants could give vent to upon seeing themselves excluded from the places of honor during the ceremony.

One more battle had to be waged. Whatever the nature of the generational materials contributed by male and female, generation could be reduced, in theory, to either of two possible mechanisms. In one, the progenitors contribute formless matter, which is gradually sculpted inside the mother's womb. According to this hypothesis of "epigenesis," the human conceptus starts off from a pristine substance that is progressively molded into a human infant. In the second hypothesis, of "preformation," the human embryo is already constituted whole in the seed, and all it needs is nourishment and growth to become self-sustaining. Defenders of epigenesis made much of Aristotelian metaphors. Though seasoned in Christian dressings to smother all flavor of paganism, their lucubrations repeat Aristotle's concept of "form" becoming imprinted on some sort of primeval matter. But the discovery of the concrete nature of sperm routs the supporters of epigenesis and infuses new vigor in its foes, the advocates of preformation. Religion had proclaimed that in the loins of Adam and Eve lay the seed for all future human descendance, for all generations to come. Now, the astounding discovery in sperm of millions of diminutive beings "swimming, like eels, head in front," rekindles the enthusiasm of preformationists. In the intoxicating buoyancy of this discovery, observers persuade themselves that these tailed living creatures are but means of conveyance for tiny human infants. They affirm, and no doubt believe, that behind the delicate external membrane of each one of these myriad tailed creatures one can see a miniature human infant. Crouched, wadded, balled up and tightly bent, in fetal position, waiting only for the right environment in which to shed the external wrapping, there to grow to human scale. It thus warms the hearts of pious microscopists to confirm that the progress of man's knowledge constantly reaffirms the revealed truths of the faith. For it is true that man carries within his body the seed for all generations to come, throughout all centuries, till the end of the human race.

Even as it seemed most assured, however, the preformationists' triumph was vitiated by doubt. If the male, in fact, delivers a living creature with all its component parts into the maternal womb, one must perforce grant that this living creature contains, in turn, the germ of its own offspring. But this offspring, to be complete, must house its own offspring; and so on, in endless succession. Preformationism proposes a biology of *"emboîtement"*—that is, of the boxing-in of generations. François Jacob calls it the "Russian-doll hypothesis,"[2] since it posits that one human being carries a smaller one inside, and the latter a still smaller one, and so forth. Now, the microscope had shown that the size ratio between an adult man and one of his sperm cells (within which, presumably, travels his complete, tiny offspring) was approximately $1/1,000,000,000$. That is, an adult man is one thousand million times bigger than one of his sperm cells. Buffon carries the argument to its logical conclusion in his *Histoire naturelle des animaux*. The ratio between a man and the germ of his own son is "expressed by a number of ten digits." But if we consider the germ of the second generation, the ratio becomes a number of nineteen digits. For our great-grandsons, the ratio is one of twenty-seven digits. The size of the germ for our heirs down to the sixth generation would be expressed by a denominator of fifty-four digits. Now, if it is true that Adam's loins contained the seed for all humanity down through the ages, we would have to believe that he harbored a seed-within-a-seed that in only six generations was already infinitesimally smaller than the smallest particle visible with the most powerful microscope. As to the seed for our own selves, removed far more than six generations from Adam, it must have been so very tiny that to represent it with numbers we would have to use figures many times larger than those used by astronomers to measure the total span of the known universe. Who would believe this in the heyday of rationalism?

Thus, the partisans of epigenesis take heart. Preformation is impossible. It must be, then, that human beings develop out of some kind of ductile substratum, which is gradually shaped into a human being. What this substance may be, and what the forces that shape it, are problems to be faced later, as knowledge advances. In the meantime, it is necessary to accept the existence of this pristine matter, from which the fetus is fashioned out. But this implies an inherent plasticity in the substratum that ought not to be disregarded by the true philosopher. The brightest minds of the Enlightenment had ruled out an influence of extraneous causes, such as the mother's emotions, on the bodily conformation of the fetus. The problem must now be reexamined, though with greater caution, to avoid former fallacies. In the long span of nine months many are the objects that present themselves to the mother. Many that are capable of moving her, horrifying her, kindling her appetites, or otherwise provoking a strong commotion in her brain. It is easy, but fallacious, to find in this or that feature of the fetus a corroboration of one's belief in the formative power of the maternal imagination. A mother reports having sat, while pregnant, under a cherry tree from which a large number of cherries suddenly dropped to the ground. Subsequently, she gave birth to an infant covered by a large number of cherry-red excrescences. These were probably the common vascular tumors called hemangiomas, but the temporal sequence of the occurrences tempts the observer to adjudicate the first one the cause, and the second one the effect, "for," writes the learned Father Benito Jerónimo Feijóo y Montenegro, "this form of bastard threading is the logic that rules the world." Nor is the vehemence of the impression a sufficient cause of corporeal deformation of the fetus. Torture of criminals in public, notes our Father, is often witnessed by pregnant women, many of whom are squeamish and soft-hearted. Execution by hanging provokes in all who witness it a deep, strange perturbation of the soul. How is it, then, that infants are never born with a compressed neck, a violaceous, swollen face, or a protruding tongue? All of which shows that one should never be too quick to attribute formative influences to the mother's emotions. Nonetheless, since the fetus is not delivered whole into the womb, and since it seems to be formed out of a material that must be inordinately plastic, prudence counsels us not to deny intransigently all influence to extraneous causes. A middle ground is recommended by the thoughtful: the maternal imagination can leave its impress on the fetus if it is active during the moment of conception, but not thereafter. Feijóo had an opportunity to apply this principle when he was confronted by the following problem of genetics, on which he was consulted. In the village of Marchena, distant nine miles from Seville, a nobleman named Francisco de Ahumada had been born with the somatic features of the black race, or as it was said then, "Ethiopian." His hair was frizzy, his nose was broad, and the color of his skin altogether "Ethiopian." However, both his father and mother were of a perfect whiteness, and the illustrious line of descent of this family made an illicit commerce of the mother with an Ethiopian slave an unthinkable (and unsafe) conjecture. But, most remarkable circumstance, the two brothers of the study case ("the propositus" is the modern term) were white. One of them, don Isidro, was blond and blue-eyed; the other one, don Antonio, was white without reaching these extremes of hypopigmentation. All possibilities were discussed, in a show of scientific objectivity. A culpable union of the mother was ruled out because the offspring of black father and white mother is mulatto, whereas don Francisco's perfect blackness was unquestioned. Moreover, his descendance was mulatto. An in-field investigation in the Ahumada's homestead promptly raised the data requisite for a tenable hypothesis. In the bed-chamber where the Ahumada successors had been conceived, there were a number of oil paintings of religious subjects. Conspicuous among them was one representing the Adoration of the Magi. What, if not the spectacle of the three wise men from the East, had caused the peculiar range of color in the three heirs of the Ahumada family? As to don Francisco's blackness, "to what other cause could it obey, if not to the vehement imagination of the mother clinging to the semblance of the Black Magus at the moment of conception?"[3]

It is not generally known that the discovery of the role of spermatozoa in fertilization is a very recent development. It is attributed to Rudolph A. von Kölliker (1817–1905) in the late nineteenth century. Throughout most of the last century the old views on the lack of significance of spermatozoa in generation continued to be reiterated: They are not animal forms. It is not sufficient, to include them in the animal kingdom, that they move. Animals have mobility, but they also reproduce and digest. Sperm cells have never been known to accomplish these functions, thus they are "free vibratile threads." They are no more animals than "the pollen that fertilizes plants." (They are plants!) On the other hand, some investigators assent to the claims that the sperm cells may be animal forms, but they classify them together with protozoa found in ponds and stagnant water, as if to emphasize their role as adventitious "contaminants." Czermak classifies them with infusoria. And the preformationist conception has not died out yet. Valentin, studying the sperm of a bear, convinced himself that he could see in sperm cells the outline of a proboscis, a stomach, and even intestinal convolutions. But by the late nineteenth century sperm cells are being examined by the implacable light of positivism and experimentation. Nothing, in the awesome biologic function of generation, is sacred any more. The mysteries of this function are trivialized. Wishing for popularity and success, a French physician wrote a book on the pathology and physiology of sex. It is a book of popular divulgation, but it summarized all that was known about sperm in 1899.[4] The author lists what salts and chemical compounds remain after its evaporation; what techniques best stain the sperm cells for microscopic examination; what the effect is of lowering temperature on the mobility of spermatozoa; how many are present in each ejaculate; what the speed of their displacement under different environmental conditions is; how their mobility is affected by warming one end and cooling the opposite end of the glass slide on which they are examined. And together with all these data come statements that remind us that the Age of Innocence is not altogether in the past. The description of sperm starts this way: "The sperm liquid is heavier than water, viscous, stringy, and has a special odor, compared by some to that of grated horn, but rather, in our opinion, to that of the first bloom of the chestnut tree." While recounting the experiences of physiologists who discovered that the zoosperms were still alive twenty-four or more hours after the death of guillotined men, a Parisian *fin-de-siècle* playfulness intrudes into the narrative. If viable sperm cells can thus retain their vitality, they could be transported across long distances in bottles, without loss of inseminating potency. Children sired by these means could be called "escapees from the bottle," just like the genii in the *Thousand and One Nights.* And what a subject for a farce! Imagine Mr. A, away from home, enlisted in the army, and wishing to inseminate Mrs. A, who has remained back home, on account of his fear of dying in battle without leaving descendants. Imagine, next, Mr. B wishing to do the same with Mrs. B. Both husbands mail their bottled semen to their respective wives. However, a confusion of packages takes place in the post office, as a result of which Mr. A's bottled seminal fluid is applied to Mrs. B, and Mr. B's to Mrs. A. In the epilogue of this farce, for which the title "Escaped from the Bottle, or Adultery by Post" is suggested, the plaintiff husbands bring a legal suit of paternity against the postmaster general.

Less than a century later, our knowledge of the biology of generation has surpassed the mischievous speculations of the Parisian doctor. "Escapees from the bottle" are a reality, customarily referred to in the news media as "test-tube babies." But our technological prowess produces no farces; rather, it raises serious—dead serious—issues. Legal suits are brought, not against the postmaster general, but against physicians and technologists who perform procedures that result in a "wrongful birth." This is the strange new legal term[5,6] first recognized by the courts of the United States in 1967, when the decision was made that, under certain circumstances, being conceived constitutes an injury entitling the concerned parties (the individual born, and/or the parents) to redress. Adults have sued physicians when conception followed an ineffective surgical operation performed to curtail fertility. Parents of a child born with serious malformations or incurable disease also seek compensation under the "wrongful birth" cause of legal action. The courts, in general, refuse to admit that what is at issue is the right *not* to be born. Metaphysical questions have never made for clearness in any field, least of all in law. Thus, whether it might have been better never to have been born than to be born with serious and irreparable physical impairments is something that judges will not worry about. Neither will they face the question of whether the parents' emotional suffering from conceiving an "unwanted" or physically defective child is balanced or outweighed by the feelings of love that parenthood brings along. But within the last five or six years, more and more American courts, to the dismay of the professionals that stand to become targets of these legal actions, feel inclined to grant compensation for damages resulting from "wrongful births." Implied in these rulings is the conviction that the mysteries of genetic impairment have utterly ceased to be such; that we possess sufficient knowledge to give us certainty as to what the outcome will be in many gestations; and that we are equipped with the technology necessary to prevent generation-associated catastrophes.

Clearly, the history of human generation has reached the crossroads. The enormous success of this biologic function, joined to an increasing ability to control disease and premature death, has overpopulated the earth. After centuries of stability, the world's population reached 700 million in 1750, 1 billion in 1850, 2 billion in 1930, and is nearly 4 billion today. The United Nations projection (which assumes a constant fertility) is for 7,522 million, or close to 8 billion, by the year 2000.[7] This avalanche of humanity was produced by no other expedient than that of following the natural biologic urge of heterosexual coupling. (Parenthetically, this statement in no way implies condonation of the epithet "anti-natural" for homosexual pairing. The liberal, enlightened stance of official medicine in our day seems to comprehend at last the viewpoint of the homosexual minority, well summed up in an old Italian story long before the official pronouncement of American psychiatrists. A fisherman suspected of homosexual activity, asked at confession if he had sinned *contra natura*, denied all with conviction. Later, faced with the incriminating evidence, he candidly admitted: "Ah! I was asked whether I had sinned against nature. But, to me, the desire for boys comes as naturally as that for food and drink.") Heterosexual mating, practiced with the millenarian spontaneity of unimpeded biology, has overcrowded the globe. All former stratagems by which men and women contrived to deflect, promote, or somehow modify generation counted for little. Their contriving makes for interesting or amusing stories, but, in the aggregate, had no visible impact on the designs of nature. It is otherwise in our times. The wherewithal is at hand by which human generation is to experience profound, worldwide modifications. And the willingness to use it, at least in the industrialized countries, is no longer in doubt. The conscientious National Fertility Study (NFS) showed that by 1970, more than one out of every five married women of reproductive age in the United States were using oral contraceptives; of "older" couples between 30 and 44 years of age, one quarter had resorted to permanent measures of sterilization, such as tubal ligation for the wife or vasectomy for the husband.[8] Only 15 percent of the couples investigated reported never having used anticonceptive measures, and according to NFS researchers, the principal reasons for non-use were "ignorance, indifference, or lowness in conceiving." Religious persuasion had virtually no influence, since the proportion of Catholic women between 18 and 39 years of age who use these contraceptive technics (i.e., other than the rhythm method) increased from 30 percent in 1955 to 68 percent in 1970. It seems that contemporary women have made a firm decision. The Grand Duke of Tuscany's injunction to the Queen of France, *Fate figliuoli in ogni modo* ("Make babies any way you can"), is interpreted in reverse—avoid them any way you can—by most women in industrialized societies.

There is no evidence that mankind has taken a sudden dislike for generational activities. To judge from the overenthusiastic participation of men and women in these proceedings, one would guess that generation enjoys an all-time popularity. The difference is that generation is no longer to flow spontaneously: it is to be foreseen, pre-planned, guaranteed for freedom from deficiencies. At least in the industrialized countries, we mean to control it, and the first step in this control has been to decrease it. The governments of all developed countries acknowledge as much. For instance, the Council on Environmental Quality of the United States recently stated that a further decline in fertility is expected in this country,[9] as a result of the generalized desire to limit the size of families. It is not difficult to predict that the use of contraceptive methods will increase. The massive clinical experience already attained, and the urgency of further scientific research made necessary by widespread use, indicate that contraceptives soon will reach a nearly "perfect" state, pharmacologically speaking. Contraceptive agents will become one hundred per cent effective, low in cost, easily prepared, with virtually no untoward effects even after prolonged use or sudden discontinuation; they will reach even wider distribution and easier availability than they now have; possibly, some will be usable by men as well as women. All this will happen first in the industrialized countries; their peoples, placed ahead in the race for those tantalizing, unseizable rewards that our imagination ciphers out as "happiness," will be the first ones to experience complete dominion over generation. Already enjoying unprecedented material comfort, they are now receiving the freedom to choose whether their offspring is to be or not to be. There is nothing like this in the historical past, or in the distressing present in large areas of the world. Two were the secular sustaining axes of the remarkably circular path of the lives of millions of people: material want and generation. A lady of the court of Louis XIV reprimanded a poor young woman who dragged three grimy children while carrying an infant in her arms, and admonished her to stop conceiving infants that she could not feed. To which the young woman replied: "What did you expect? When we are without bread, we throw ourselves upon the meat-flesh." Modern man will renounce neither. The contemporary idea of happiness is some kind of bread-and-meat concoction, like a quiche Lorraine.

Birth control, however, is only the beginning. We would have generation control in the broad sense. For the reason that, make no mistake, we can do it. The Huxleyian Brave New World, in which an unfeeling bureaucracy decides who is born and who is not, and prescribes the predetermined traits that the offspring is to have in order to best serve the interests of those in power, is not here yet. But the hints of its earliest beginnings are unmistakable. Techniques are already available that enable us to choose the sex of the unborn. Sperm cells carry either the X chromosome, which produces girls, or the Y chromosome, which produces boys. Because the X chromosome is bigger and heavier, girl-producing sperm cells can be separated from boy-producing sperm cells by techniques using centrifugation, or gel-filtration methods, without loss of inseminating potency.[10] These procedures are still fraught with technical difficulties that interfere with their general application, and which it falls beyond our present scope to discuss here. Nevertheless, the know-how that makes such sex selection possible is already here. Ardent controversy, therefore, has already started. The debate is about what no one has seen yet, and thus it has a little of the ring, and to my mind the charm, of the debates of the schoolmen in the Middle Ages. The main arguments have appeared in hundreds of articles in specialized journals of various disciplines; some are summarized in what follows. The interested reader is referred to a recently published book devoted to the problems attending sex selection.[11]

What if parents could choose with minimal inconvenience—say, by taking a pill in the morning—the sex of their child? Optimists say that this would be a boon; that, where sex is concerned, there would be no more "wrongful births," since every child would be a "wanted child." Parents would be contented and satisfied. It is true that an extra supply of boys would be engendered, because scientists have shown that throughout the world the number of parents wishing for boys greatly exceeds those who want girls. But this imbalance, the optimist party says, would be a good thing, too. It would tend to offset the present excess of women, thus decreasing the amount of loneliness and alienated spinsterhood to which many women are condemned in their mature years. Lastly, and this is perhaps the decisive argument wielded by the optimist faction, the ability to generate boys at will would alleviate the world's overpopulation. This reasoning is two-pronged. Firstly, many families today, especially in the Third World, base their fecundity on the "gambler's fallacy": they keep having children if the first few births are productive of girls, thinking that the odds are greater of having a boy with each successive pregnancy (they are not: the odds are fifty-fifty each time). In many societies, the birth of boys is not merely a question of pride and social prestige —themselves powerful motivating forces—but also a genuine economic preoccupation. Girls often represent a liability for the financial resources of the family; parents expect to compensate this potential risk by generating boys, the providers of income and security in old age. Therefore, the conclusion is that the family size would be limited if progenitors could have the certainty of getting a boy on a first try, and would abandon their current tendency to "try again" after one or more girl-producing attempts. Secondly, in a society with a greatly decreased number of women the opportunities for a true population explosion are limited. Unlike men, women must carry the child for the duration of gestation, and during this period no new pregnancies are possible. As a researcher colorfully explained: "the rate-limiting factor in population growth [is] the number of uteruses."[12]

For each one of these arguments, however, a contrary proposition may be adduced. To imagine that parental frustration would entirely cease upon the birth of a "wanted" child is to manifest a naive conception of the springs that move the human heart. Restlessness and dissatisfaction are the perpetual lot of all but the blessed few. To bring a new, independent, self-willed being into the world is hardly a way to ensure that one's hopes will not be thwarted. In this sense, parenthood always means, by its very nature, greater or lesser degrees of disappointment. For it is not to be assumed that parenthood strengthens the fitful or sobers the immature. Nor is it in the sex of the offspring, but in its achievements, qualities, and filial sentiments, that parents find whatever gratification may attach itself to parenting. And if it is argued that worldly achievement is easier for males, the obvious answer is that what must then be corrected is not the sex of the unborn, but the social injustice that permits an unequal treatment of the sexes. To do any less is to condone tacitly the perpetuation of an iniquitous system that favors men over women regardless of their individual merits and qualifications. This is a premise that may be predicated on purely egalitarian grounds, yet an important practical consequence of it would be to dampen population growth, because the insistence on having boys by repeated pregnancies is likely to be modified in a society where equal opportunities are tendered to individuals of one or the other sex. As to the relief of forlorn widows and dejected spinsters, it must be remembered that the problem is largely a consequence of women's longer life span;[13] this being so, it is an unfair solution to seek a remedy in an oversupply of men. A more equitable and humanitarian solution would be to endeavor to prolong men's lives. There is a shortage of companions for mature and elderly women, but this should not be regarded from a fatalistic vantage point. Rather, we ought to take into account the fact that the scarcity of men issues from the attrition that comes with the stressful manner of life to which men subject themselves in payment for social advancement and success. Public-health measures that promote men's welfare are attentive to women's needs only in a roundabout way, but their implementation is likely to enjoy the cooperation of most men. And even if some women doubt the validity of this reasoning, they would do well to ponder on the consequences of living in a world overstocked with men. From historical experience they ought to know that when their fates lay entirely in men's hands, men did not always feel disposed to treat them fairly. Once they become vastly outnumbered by men, there is no guarantee that reality will conform to their expectations. Instead of an increased freedom to pick and choose, they may well encounter a multiplied number of oppressors. Or, to use the Oriental metaphors that have been so effectively used by sociologists debating this topic, instead of the male harem of which they dream, they could get purdah.[12]

How would it feel to live in a world in which the proportion of men greatly exceeded that of women? Some claim that such a world would usher in irreparable social dislocations. To women is owed much of the benign and refined tone that tempers the harshness in the collective struggle for survival. Women read more books, support more charitable and philanthropic institutions than do men. Patrons of the arts are apt to be patronesses. Women attend readings of poetry and ballet performances, and generally abet cultural endeavors that, without their sponsorship, would wane. With a decreased feminine presence, would the life of societies take on some of the air of the military barracks? Considering that competition for females would become fiercer, and that men's aggressiveness on this score can be frightful, would social violence reach heights greater than any previously known? The nature of the relationship between men and women would certainly change. It seems unlikely that this relationship would become less conflictive in the future world anticipated by some social scientists. And the family would also change in unpredictable ways. Few children would know the experience of being reared with an older sister, since most first-borns would be boys. Hence, the psychology of the individuals composing the new society would be altered in subtle and unforeseeable ways. They would be predominantly a generation of male first-borns interacting with other male first-borns, and thus shaping their personalities through experiences of lasting influence, but whose precise nature we cannot ascertain. All these speculations, though idle at the present hour, show that interference with the natural world is a much more complex undertaking than is commonly surmised. All things in the world are connected as if by subtle threads, and it is useless to think that one piece may be suddenly jarred without making the others shake. Lack of appreciation of the extended consequences of our modifications of nature's plans can lead to disastrous results. Ecologic devastation is perhaps the glaring example, for it may be said of modern societies what Tacitus said of the Romans: "they make a desert, and they call it peace." It would not be superfluous to pause and reflect before tampering with a sex ratio that, in the course of thousands of years, nature produced in the human species through free and unhampered genetic interplay.[14]

Well into the pathway of mass contraception, modern societies would be well advised to pause and ask questions before taking the next step. I believe it is not entirely useless to ask whether the newly acquired control over generation has made men and women happier. The answer, in my view, is not to be found in the discussions of sociologists and anthropologists. Certainly not in the literature of scientists responsible for the advancement of genetic engineering. Not even in the writings of serious philosophers meditating on the ethical consequences of scientific progress in this field. Here we must turn to novelists, whose observations may not influence public policy, but who can give us a close view of the beats of individual human hearts. In a remarkable recent novel by Günter Grass, *Headbirths, Or The Germans Are Dying Out,* the writer offers us, among other striking and original insights, a glimpse of the personal problems of a childless middle-class couple in contemporary West Germany. They are both teachers in secondary school. They are both veterans of the student protest movement, socially conscious, introspective, orderly and, it seems, systematically German at every pore. Their ambivalence over generation surfaces from the first chapter. She would like to have a child, but, on second thought, what future awaits it in an overpopulated world? He says that to become a father is "theoretically possible." But no, not now, they must wait for a better time. After the elections. After he knows what is to be done with his aging mother. Their conversations daily revolve about the "what ifs" and the "supposing thats" of pre-parenthood. On the one hand, a case could be made that to bring a new life into the world is both a duty and a joy. On the other hand, to let loose a new life into a world increasingly contaminated by radiation, a world that looks more and more like an "atomic concentration camp," is morally objectionable. In the next chapter, he accuses her of egoism, of denying him fatherhood out of her love of travel and independence. A few paragraphs later, she announces that she is going off the pill, but he points out how inconvenient it would be to have a baby now that preparations are complete for their Asian trip. Should they take an infant along in their tour of the slums of Manila? Do they vaccinate babies against cholera and yellow fever? Should they carry bags, diapers, a sterilizer for bottles, and cans of baby food to Bangkok? All right, but in any case, she wants a child. She wants a child!! As soon as they are airborne, she swears, she goes off the pill. A few lines down the narrative, as a turbaned servant in Bombay removes the dirty tableware after the couple have taken their breakfast in a hotel, she grabs a glass of water and promptly swallows the pill. Throughout the rest of this short "experimental" novel, Günter Grass juxtaposes images of primeval Asiatic fertility, of life-giving, awesome deities, to the perpetual dubiety of his German couple. Amidst the huddled, sweaty masses of the Asiatic continent, now discountenanced, now horrified, now charmed or hypnotized by the alien, exotic sights, the two characters continue their "Yes-to-baby, No-to-baby" controversy. In the last scene, back again in their hometown of Itzehoe, having resumed their work in the secondary school, the two are driving home when they narrowly miss running over a young Turkish boy in an immigrant workers' area of the town. Except for a screeching of brakes, nothing happens. Other children come to congratulate the little boy: "Now from side streets and backyards, from all directions come more and more children, all foreign. Indian, Chinese, African children, all cheerful. They fill the streets with life, wave from windows, jump from walls, innumerable. All cheer for the little Turk, who has been lucky again. They crowd around him, run their hands over him. They run their hands over the well-preserved VW where sit our childless teacher couple, not knowing what to say in German."[15]

Nothing more needs to be said. The scene accurately depicts the state of the world. The people of the developed countries, enfranchised from the acute, harrowing distress of material want, roost in their comfort and benignantly accept the gift of generational control. Everywhere else, below a line that roughly corresponds to 30° latitude north, wholesale cutting of umbilical cords is going on. In Asia, Africa and Latin America, births increase annually to the tune of three or five percent or more; babies pile up year by year, like money loaned on compound interest. But as to happiness, that prize that none of us can define but all of us think we ought to be able to attain in reasonable measure, it is nowhere to be seen. Not in the crowded tenements, and not in the house with the two-car garage. In the former, because it simply does not fit, replete as the place already is with pain, misery and disease, and crushed humanity; in the latter, because it is always being confused with something else: material affluence, technical advances, leisure, free sex, birth control, and what have you. To those inclined not to believe all this, I say: consider the last instance of its mistaken identity. We could have sworn that what lay behind the control of generation was nothing but happiness. But scarcely have we obtained the weakest empire over this function, than we realize our error. Bewilderment, confusion, anguish is what we encounter. We have barely begun to interfere with generation; at present our sophistication does not go beyond an ability to say yea or nay to this biologic function. And already we worry ourselves stiff over the consequences.

The debate continues. Some say that our desire to interfere with the workings of nature should be curtailed, because our ability to do so largely exceeds our analytical capacity to foresee the consequences. Others say that stronger and better interference is what is needed. And in the meantime, the Germans are dying out.

On Aging

Do you know, Moncrif," said Louis XV to his vassal, "that many people give you between seventy-five and eighty years of age?" "Yes, *Sire,*" was the answer, "but I am not taking them." To refuse to take the adding years; to look elsewhere, anywhere but to our own ineluctable decay: this is the head-in-the-sand strategy that we oppose to the might of nature. Nor can it be said that this is the contriving of the simple-minded, for our efforts at ignoring or concealing age range from the subtly clever to the disingenuous. Age concealment by women, tradition has it, has carried the palm. "It is terrible to grow old alone," says a contemporary joke. "My wife has not had a birthday in six years." And the feminine enthusiasm for arresting the fatal summation of years reaches at times beyond passive refusal to keep adding; it may become an active process of subtraction. Of a prominent socialite who declared herself younger and younger as the years went by, a cynical wit said that, if the trend continued, the lady would soon have to be placed under the official tutelage of her youngest daughter.

It would be false to say that men approach old age with that poised equanimity and preparedness of mind of which Epictetus spoke. It may be true, however, that women dread the coming of a certain age with far greater intensity. It takes no great powers of perception to see in this fear one more token of the unfair treatment to which they have been subjected. Forced as they are to rely, more often than men, on purely physical qualities—charm, beauty, or attractiveness—to secure a position in society, it is not surprising that they should view the imminent loss of the attributes on which so much store is placed with increasing anxiety. And unfortunately this situation of dependency persists today. Ability to found a family, status in society, and, sometimes, job security, are often subordinate, for women, to physical beauty. Consequently, there is still a panic-zone, a dreaded age at which the perceived minimal standards of freshness and vigor can no longer be maintained. The only relief that contemporary society seems to offer is a modest postponement of the dreaded age. It used to be under twenty years in the Middle Ages. In the refined court of Versailles, an "older woman" deserved this appellation at twenty-five. Courtiers of those times, wise in the ways of feminine flattery, were no strangers to exploitative manipulation of women's fears, as a story of a chronicler makes clear. A king complained that too many accidents of horse-drawn *cabriolets* were taking place on the roads next to the palace, and commanded D'Argenson to take care of the problem. This gentleman, the first appointed official in charge of city traffic, knew that *cabriolets* were the fashion of the day, and that the prettiest and most delicate hands were not always the most deft with the reins. He asked whether His Majesty wished accidents reduced in number to a more tolerable level, or suppressed altogether. The king, intrigued, answered that he wished, of course, no accidents at all in the future. D'Argenson left with a reverence and went straight to his private chamber, to write a city ordinance whereby permission to drive a horse-drawn carriage could not be issued to persons who had not reached "the age of reason," twenty-five years. The problem disappeared completely. More than a hundred years later, in czarist Russia, this eidetic scarecrow, the "dreaded age," had somewhat receded. A young princess at a ball coquettishly said to a physician who requested the next dance: "Please! Let me rest. Remember that I am a sixty-year-old lady!" The unwitting beau replied: "Bah! I have long learned to believe only half of what I hear." Whereupon, he received a slap in the face. He had guessed, it seems, a little too exactly. Today, the "dreaded age" is repulsed yet farther. Forty, forty-five, fifty or fifty-five; enthusiasm for physical fitness, lengthening of life expectancy, and generally improved living conditions allow for deferment of the day that one must enter the anxiety zone. But wherever this zone begins, make no mistake: anxiety there is, uneasiness there is, and, in some cases, sheer living terror.

Who is this frightful enemy that so strikes terror in the hearts of all, and routs even the most courageous half of mankind (women) into disorderly retreat? An imposing foe, indeed, but one that is all torpor, slowness, and parsimony. In its countenance we confirm what we all know, that it is kith and kin of death. Aging is death's cousin once removed, just as loss of consciousness or sleep is its brother. In advanced old age Saint Vincent de Paul frequently dozed off, as the elderly are wont to do, and explained his somnolence by saying: "The brother is here, with me, waiting for the sister." For the Greeks, Hypnos and Thanatos, two twins, were often conjoined. In sleep we are all alike, and so we are in death. "The sister," the brother, and the cousin share common propensities: they tend to homogenize us. Dictatorially they impose the ultimate democracy, for this is the family of the Great Levelers. Young men, said Juvenal (Sat. X, 196–201), can still be recognized as individuals: A stronger than B, B more handsome than A, ". . . but old men look all alike, all share the same bald pate. Their noses drip like an infant's, their voices tremble as much as their limbs, and they mumble their bread with toothless gums."

It is this uniformity of structure that hampered our understanding of aging. The pathology of aging easily ensnares the unwary observer. It seems natural, after looking at the bent bones, the worn-out cartilages, the thinned skin, to conclude that one sees bodily parts that have been "used up." The roughness of cartilages of sliding joints suggests that constant friction has eroded their formerly smooth, lustrous surfaces. The sturdiest structure, if rubbed, hit, burdened, and bent, day in and day out, will yield in the end; the hardest rock is worn away by the wind. Degenerative arthritis in the elderly thus appears as the mark of repeated mechanical shocks and stresses on the skeleton. Hundreds of steps are taken every day, thousands every month, and then millions over the course of years. Hence, we come to believe that the pressures of weight bearing affect the mortises and tenons of the skeletal framework. And is it not logical to propose that the heart itself fails by a similar mechanism? The calcified arteries, the hardened cardiac valves of old people seem, on but slight reflection, the obligatory consequence of the rhythmic clash of the bloodstream against them, with each pulsation of the heart, minute by minute, day by day, for all the years that it takes to become old. The sexual function is no exception. A specialist in the management of disorders associated with old age wrote that it was a common belief among many men that a limited supply of semen was made available, at birth, to each one. From this concept of "biologic entropy" issued the conviction that a man could afford a set number of ejaculations, after which he would no longer be capable of sustaining sexual relationships, at least not to the point of ejaculation.[1] Old age, therefore, appeared as something contingent, something that occurs in consequence of reiterative use of the body; related to the number of heartbeats, or to the total number of steps that we have taken, up and down, trepidating over straight and anfractuous roads.

The "wear-and-tear" concept of old age no longer rules our thinking. Unlike inanimate objects, living tissues are not wasted away *because* of reiterative use. It is precisely the opposite: lack of function produces atrophy. Disuse is a chief cause of pathology. Bones relieved of their burden become brittle, bow with greater ease than weight-bearing ones. The degeneration of immobilized joints is swifter and more severe than for those that retain a measure of their hinging action. Arteries that no longer convey the bloodstream, like all tissues whose activity is suspended, suffer irreparable damage, unless the interruption of their function be partial or transient. Our own senescence, therefore, is a much more complex phenomenon than a simple wear-and-tear. It is the expression of a detailed plan that was encoded in every one of our cells from the day we were conceived. Just as all our tissues "know" that they are to grow to a certain size, and no more, by referring to this master plan, so they are informed (or as it is fashionable to say, "programmed") to stop growing, to desist from the performance of their assigned function, and ultimately to engage in the deadly operations that will form their biologic entombment. It is therefore accurate to say that each one of us carries inside his own individual old age. We harbor within us the means of our own termination, just as we carry with us the seed, the means of our own propagation.

My professional bias has been to seek insights into the normal life processes by an attentive canvassing of deviancy. However, abnormal unfolding of the master plan of senescence is an extremely rare occurrence. Few medical professionals have had the opportunity to observe an instance of breakdown in this most meticulously respected of life processes. And yet, the revealing exemplars have long been recognized. Since 1886, when Sir Thomas Hutchison first described the disease known as *progeria*, it has been known that the speed at which the thread of life is normally spun may be altered. Victims of this disease see their lives condensed in ways that exceed the fantasy of the tales of mythology and folklore. In the first year of life the scalp thins out, the skin loses its infantile turgor. By two years of age, the prominent forehead veins, the thin, beaked nose, the shallow cheeks give the patient a wizened look, an uncanny resemblance to those oldsters that Leonardo sketched in a famous drawing. Theirs is, in the graphic (though insensitive) expression of some clinicians, a "plucked-bird appearance." At three or four years of age the joints stiffen, and arthritis becomes progressive. By the time these unfortunate infants reach the age at which healthy youths posed as models for Murillo's angels, their appearance is that of dwarfed old men: their heads balding, their joints deformed, their thin but well-proportioned limbs supporting a withered trunk of pendulous abdomen, their piping voices accentuating the impression of caricaturesque senility. If they survive to the second decade, their end is near. Autopsy studies have shown severe coronary artery disease in some of these patients as early as nine years of age. What for a normal human being is youthful eclosion, for them is terminus: they usually die in their teens, of myocardial infarction, as in old age.

Progeria does not exhaust the pathology of accelerated aging. There are other diseases that manifest at least one feature of this uncanny disobedience to biologic time. Their names are abstruse and often eponymic, as is usual for conditions of obscure origin: terms such as Werner's syndrome, Rothmund's syndrome, Cockayne's syndrome. In an international symposium on aging and cancer, held in Washington, D.C., in 1980, the disorders of accelerated aging were classified into sixteen different diseases that manifest one isolated aspect consistently associated with aging (such as premature whitening of hair or hardening of the arteries) and eleven other diseases in which a cluster of manifestations of the senile process become apparent before their time.[2] What becomes readily apparent is the extraordinary complexity of the biology of aging. Of an assumed upper limit of 100,000 genes in man, it was calculated that approximately 7,000 genes participate in the aging process. In other words, thousands of components of the genetic "blueprint" that controls life processes modulate the changes that take place in senectitude—loss of hair, eye cataracts, loss of skin turgor, degenerative changes of the heart valves, and so forth. This discouraging advice flows from belief in the preeminence of genetics in the process of aging: "If you wish to attain longevity, you must choose the right parents." But it would be untrue to claim that all is inheritance in aging. There is also the contingent. There is attrition, structural wasting away (at least of non-living bodily parts, such as teeth), cell loss and accumulation of waste products. All of this brings about life's detriment. And there are bombardment by radiation, viruses, atmospheric pollutants, deleterious life habits, and an almost endless number of potential factors contributing to senescence but whose exact role is at present unknown.

Science has a long way to go before it can hope to interfere successfully with the agenda of our internal decay. This is not to say that the ills that affect the elderly are without remedy. Medicine can do much to alleviate the concomitants of senectitude, but scientific understanding of its fundamental determinants is still rudimentary. Nor is this surprising, since gerontology is a new discipline. Strange as it seems for a phenomenon that affects us all, biologic senescence had not been approached strictly as a subject of scientific enquiry before Claude Bernard. Biologists before him (and many since) could not discard a frame of mind that inclined more to philosophical contemplation than to biologic experimentation. In *The Biology of Senescence*, Alex Comfort[3] points out that the notion that senescence is "inherent" in living matter was always accepted uncritically. "Inherent" is a term more for the philosopher than for the biologist; the latter should restrict himself to finding out what happens. Moreover, if senescence implies loss of reproductive capacity, the statement is incorrect, for it has now been shown that human cells may be maintained in culture indefinitely without losing their capacity to divide. On the other hand, our tools and properties, our friends and enemies, inanimate objects and living beings, all decay. It is thus not surprising that "generalization and analogy instead of experimentation and analysis" have dominated the thinking of researchers, even the most able. And then, aging is linked to time, and time will not be separated from metaphysics. For time has so rich a philosophical-poetical suggestiveness that few could resist engaging in speculation over its multiple dimensions; fewer yet were so prosaic as to sit down to investigate and count purely "biologic time," and nothing more. Scarcely a decade has passed since biologists first openly professed to disregard all considerations on the nature of time and its perception, and to be concerned simply with what exactly happens when an organism ages. And already a new discipline, "chronobiology," has emerged. Attention is focused on the "internal clock," free at last from the shackles of all subjective considerations. We begin to learn how the body keeps its own rhythmicity: cells from various organs divide following daily or nightly mitotic bursts; the internal glands secrete their hormones with periodic rises and falls; susceptibility to certain drugs varies with the hour of the clock. And much of this activity is free from environmental influences: our body "knows" its individual, biologic time, maintained for long periods in the dark. In consequence, much of what we thought we had learned must now be relearned. When we say that a given substance exists in the body at x concentration, do we mean in the morning or at night, or are we speaking of an average value? And if the values fluctuate, how and why is the rhythm modified with the advance of age? All of which reiterates the humbling complexity, the devilish intricacy that underlies the mechanisms of senescence.

Seen in this light, efforts to forestall the progress of senescence appear disarmingly naive. But many respected researchers, as opposed to quacks, mystics, and eccentrics, have labored with this goal in mind. Brown-Séquard was convinced that testicular extracts had a rejuvenating effect (1899); Metchnikoff viewed aging as the result of accumulation of intestinal toxins (1907), and recommended a diet rich in *Lactobacillus bulgaricus;* Voronof, of more recent memory (1929), grafted glands of nonhuman primates into aging human beings.[4] Very recently, Aslan, of Rumania, claimed a rejuvenating effect for his treatment of injections of a procaine solution, to which he gave the high-sounding name Gerovital.[5] And as late as 1975, gerontologists pleaded for controlled trials of this treatment in North America. Confirmation of the efficacy of these treatments has not been forthcoming, although perhaps the future will vindicate the partial theoretical truths in their conceptual base.

For the moment, their individual bias intrigues the curious: it is remarkable that while some have seen senescence as the outcome of dysfunction of the alimentary tract or the immunological system, others have thought that the genital system exerts the predominant control. How this notion came into being, I cannot say, for in many biologic species sexual activity effects, if anything, a shortening of the life span. The life of *Drosophila*, the fruit fly, for instance, is made shorter by copulation or egg-laying, whereas the female's life span is increased by sterilization. The picture is not so clear-cut for human beings. Often-quoted population statistics show that Catholic priests, who practice celibacy, live less long, on the average, than Protestant ministers, who marry. But caution should be exerted in interpreting these figures; a great many variables intervene which, if ignored, can prompt the wrong conclusions. Yet the popular notion persists throughout the world that something in the sexual domain of our physiology has the power to alter the rate of man's decline (not always, I might add, in the desired direction). This is what gave rise to the magic practice of *shunammitism*, the belief that an old man derives great benefit from the physical proximity of a young woman. This treatment works only for men; also, shunammitism speaks of proximity, and proximity only. Anything else could be attempted, I suppose, only at the patient's great peril. In this context, Comfort cites experimental work in rodents that shows that introduction of a young female into a colony of aging inbred males actually prolongs the life of the latter; next, we are referred to the work of the Dutch physician Boerhaave (1668–1738), who advised an old Burgomaster of Amsterdam, pining under the ills of old age, "to lie between two young girls, assuring him that he would thus recover strength and spirits." One wonders if Comfort's juxtaposition of modern experimental data and ancient magical notions was meant as a subtle suggestion that, considering the perdurability of unverified magical concepts, these ideas ought to be tested with the contemporary tools and methods of science. Christopher William Hufeland, private physician and friend of Goethe,

Schiller, and Herder, hailed today as an early pioneer of "chronobiology," remarked of shunammitism: "We cannot refuse our approval to the method." I bring it to the attention of the authorities at the National Institutes of Health that these words were spoken by someone who is now ranked as a visionary; should they wish to give consideration to the proposal, some of us may look forward, as old age sets in, to experiences less smarting than the monthly reception of a lean pensioner's check.

Our understanding of the biology of aging is thus sadly incomplete, and understanding is yet the best defense. Of course, faced with a threat, we have other options: we may choose to ignore it, or we may delude ourselves into thinking that we have adequate protection when, in fact, our shield is illusory. Both expedients are unsatisfactory. They make us look ridiculous, obtuse, or imperceptive of our needs and those of others. In one case we continue to act, to talk, to dress as if we were young, until the discrepancy between youthful dress and wrinkles, or grey beard, borders on the obscene. We rationalize the signs and symptoms: decreased physical endurance is due to indigestion, to tight clothes, to humidity in the air. Autosuggestion may be quite successful, at least for a time. I read in Tallemant de Réaux this sublime rationalization for decreased sexual potency, voiced by a peasant of Saintonge who bragged about enhanced penile strength with the passing of years: ". . . proof of this is that when I was young, I could make it function by myself whenever I wanted without any help, whereas now my wife and I, joining our efforts, can rarely succeed in imposing our will." There are less comical aspects to our delusions. We become intolerant of those less fortunate than ourselves. Ignorant of the mechanisms underlying senescence, we apply our own inflexible standards to whoever is weaker; anyone who has become helpless or dependent, we declare, bears total responsibility for his misfortune. We sermonize, we adjure. Heaven help us, we presume to condemn; callously we confuse pathology with lack of strong interests, wrongly believing that physiological decline can always be deflected by interesting hobbies.

It is difficult to disagree with the humorist who wrote: "I have discovered that men who were dull and dissatisfied when young are dull and dissatisfied when old, only more so." Conversely, the example of men and women passionately involved in their favorite activities until a ripe old age is always edifying. We think of Nicias, the painter mentioned by Plutarch, so delighted in his work that he had to ask his servants whether he had washed, or dined; of Canus, the flute player, who took so great a pleasure in his music that he averred that his audience should ask of him to pay, rather than give him money, if they only knew how much he enjoyed each performance. This anecdote of Archimedes' old age has survived: utterly absorbed in his problems of geometry, he must be plucked by force from the table on which he traces his figures, carried, lifted off the ground by his attendants and stripped of his clothes in order to be anointed, and all the while he continues to trace figures with his fingers on his anointed body. Can this intensity of involvement be without effect on physiology? It seems capable of suspending the deathward flow of life. But basic science passes no pronouncement: the effect of artistic or intellectual occupations on longevity, depending on too many uncontrollable variables, is not a subject of study. The practical branches of medicine take the view that, if certain phenomena do not lend themselves to investigation, it does not follow that their effect is insignificant. Medicine's ultimate concern is the welfare of the patient; it matters little that the bodily effect of some activities cannot be fathomed, what counts is that they do us good. It is on this account that cultivation of the arts is sanctioned as "recreational therapy." However, the effect of this therapy is a function both of previous training and innate esthetic sensibility. The soul must be in tune, as Milton said, with art, if art is to be therapeutic. Total absorption in the arts, to the point of setting us free from the cares of aging, cannot be expected in more than the fortunate few. Berlioz, like a few other musicians, sailed through life attentive more to his inner harmonies than to any external tribulation. How little affected he was by occurrences that others view as cataclysms may be inferred from his last words, when he is already in the throes of the death agony: "At last, my friend!" he was heard to say. "Now they are *really* going to play my music!" It is quite evident that a passion of this magnitude is as sturdy a defense against life's blows as one could ever hope for. But it is also evident that it is a rare gift, a dispensation, and not simply the result of training. However much others may wish to secure the gift for themselves, industry will not supply what nature has not provided. Confronting Dryden's question, "What passion cannot music raise or quell?" Jackson of Exeter sarcastically commented: "What passion *can* music raise or quell?" Clearly, an interest in art cannot be made into a universally effective prescription against the hard goings of old age.

I confess to having believed in the consolations of philosophy with all the ardor of youthful credulity. With what unforgettable emotion I read, in my youth, the pages of Epicurus, Seneca and Epictetus! Here was wisdom prepackaged and ready to be carried home, so to speak, by the determined customer. For I shared the delusion that one may place an order for wisdom in the local bookshop; that just as the hungry place an order for pizza, so do the seekers after wisdom line up at the bookshop with equal prospects of satisfaction. And this idea was reinforced by the lapidary directness of the Greek and Roman philosophers. For theirs was the language of the common man, addressed to common men, free from the jargon and pedantry with which philosophy was later gaudily dressed when she, too, aged and turned into the withered, cynical and somewhat perverse matron that she now appears to be. Would I be able to overcome despair when I became overwhelmed by weakness and old age? All I had to do was to reread those magnificent paragraphs: "It is only animality, dead weight, vice and the organs of vice, that become old. The soul is in full vigor, and congratulates itself on having less commerce with the body, for in decreasing such dealings it gets rid, at last, of a good part of its load." Would I not believe it a great pity to see myself gradually diminished, exhausted day by day, melting away by degrees and fully conscious of my doom? For consolation I would turn to Seneca, and would hear him say that there is no better exit from life than the soft declivity offered by nature to those who become very old. "Preferable," he says, "to a sudden, precipitous fall from the high point of one's full powers." It is better to descend at a stately and slow pace, leisurely contemplating our past progress, raking with our eyes the whole compass of our pilgrimage. But would I experience much pain when entering the last stages of corporeal disintegration? No: the soul of old people hangs tenuously from their lips, ready to take flight, and detaches itself therefrom without violence. "The fire ignited in a flammable stuff can only be extinguished by throwing on it much water, with great effort and usually at high cost. But when no fuel was present, the flames are easily put off, and often disappear of themselves." But how would I be able to maintain an even temper when my body could no longer be supported, like a ruinous building in which every wall cracks, where no sooner is one fissure filled with cement than another one opens up? Even these grim prospects can be faced with a smile. This, say the ancient philosophers, is what philosophy can do. It can infuse the sufferer with forbearance and courage to the very end. Nay, it increases the joyous valor as the end approaches ". . . as it is seen that the enthusiasm of runners in the stadium heightens as they enter the last lap and feel themselves coming closer to the crown of laurel."

All this worked marvelously when I was young. And even today, I cannot reread those pages without a unique delectation. But it is clear that delectation is not consolation. When the Stoics state that life is given to us with the condition that it must be ended, and that it is madness to despair because we are not made the exception to the universal rule, I am compelled to agree that they make eminently good sense. But as soon as I put down the book, I think it is a shame that all my physical vigor must fatally ebb. When the philosophers enjoin us to remain calm and untroubled in the face of occurrences that are inevitable, universal, and out of our control, I am the first to proclaim that this is the very essence of wisdom. But as soon as the book is reshelved I am overpowered by sadness in considering that old age is inevitable, death universal, and gradual enfeeblement out of our control. As to the examples of the invulnerability of wisdom, of which the Stoics furnish a voluminous and touching literature, I am moved to the innermost depth of my heart, and then I own myself incapable of emulating their example. When Demetrius had taken the city of Megara, he asked a philosopher of the captured city whether he reckoned to have lost anything. "Nothing," was the answer, "for all my things I carry with me." And it is to be noted, says Seneca, that his household had just been looted, his wife killed, his two daughters ravished, and his homeland put under the rule of foreigners; and the king questioned him from the height of his triumphal chariot, surrounded by his armed guard. Adds Seneca: "But he snatched victory from the king's hands, and in a conquered city not only was he unhurt, but he overmastered. He seized and kept the true goods, those that cannot be taken away, whereas those that had been stolen and dissipated he considered not truly his, but the adventitious bounty of Fortune. Hence he did not love them as his own, for the possession of externals is always fragile and insecure."

Now, I confess that while I read, all this keeps me entranced and in the extremity of admiration both for the sonorous style of Seneca and for the spiritual strength of the Stoic philosophers. On the other hand, as soon as the book is closed, I begin to wonder what was wrong with that philosopher of Megara. For, it seems to me, it takes an inordinate amount of insensitivity, coldness of affect, and unadulterated chutzpah to live many years with a woman, to father two daughters, and then to say that one should never really love any of them as one's own, but that the philosophically correct attitude is to relegate them to the position of adventitious, insecure gifts of volatile Fortune. In this, the Stoics are not far away from the religious mystics who followed and with whom they share an almost invincible difficulty in attracting a sincere mass following.

The lofty pronouncements of philosophy are no consolation. Cultivation of a philosophical habit of mind is one of the most delectable activities open to us. But this cultivation requires energy, and energy is gradually drained from us. Nor is it to be forgotten that there is a pathology of aging, seemingly independent of personal habits. There *is* such a thing as Alzheimer's disease, or senile dementia, and there *are* degrees of severity of this disease, and others like it, that may go unrecognized. Let us not presume to reprimand the old and infirm for lacking cultural interests to sustain them. Until more is known about the effects of age on the human brain, to accuse senile persons of improvidence is a refined form of cruelty; it is adding insult to grievous and obscure injury. Can we really expect a forward look, passionate attachment to a cause, intellectual pursuits, or social commitment of a man who cannot complete a long sentence because he has forgotten its beginning? The first step in our response to this tragedy should be to suspend all judgment. We must ascertain the mechanism of cerebral dysfunction, and why aged individuals are so differently affected, before we can claim that abject physiological decline could have been averted "if only" strong interests had been cultivated. Moreover, assuming a minimum of cerebral integrity, it remains dubious that purely intellectual interests afford the sought-after consolation. At least for philosophy, this soothing effect can be disclaimed. Nowhere is the gap between theory and practice more ludicrous than in this most exalted of intellectual disciplines; initiates are pleasantly instructed, often edified, but rarely set at peace. Nicolas Berdayev, Russian metaphysician, was once speaking passionately about the insignificance and unreality of time. To the surprise of his enthralled listeners, he stopped suddenly, in the middle of his eloquent exposition, drew out his watch, and anxiously looked at it: he was terrified of being a few minutes late in taking his medicine.

Clearly, philosophy is for the strong, who hardly need it. The enfeebled, the sick, the disconsolate, and the aged who look for a source of strength outside themselves have rarely found it in the consolations of philosophy. Religion is another line of defense. To some, religious or mystical persuasion is quite enough. But a large part, if not the majority, of mankind fail to be so fortunate. In many people, notwithstanding their fervid professions, religious belief fails to filter through all the layers of the mind. Sometimes it stops at the superficial strata of strictly conscious thought, underneath which thrives the gnawing doubt that, after all, the central belief may be erroneous or misguided. Thus, to the certainty of their bodily breakdown is added the cruel (though unvoiced) suspicion that what made tolerable this piece-by-piece depredation may itself be uncertain. For the contemplation of the gradual ruin of the body that we inhabit is made bearable by the conviction that what awaits us after the ruin is complete is "a building from God, a house not made by human hands, eternal in the heavens" (2 Cor. 5:1); and to realize the ineluctability of life's destruction, while at the same time losing all hope for some kind of eventual restitution, is a double blow harsher than many people can stand. Nor can it be said that the soothing notion of a happy immortality is a Christian idea. Fear of our own dissolution, and the sense of its imminence that comes with old age, have always been countered with a blind, visceral, almost furious will to believe in some kind of perdurability of a conscious post-self; and pagans were as prone to experience this yearning as are Christians. With this difference, that, generally speaking, pagans were more candid, and invariably more elegant, in giving voice to this desire. Cicero defined with unsurpassed lucidity the nature of this yearning when he made the aged Cato say: "If I err in this, in believing that the souls of men are immortal, I gladly err. And while I live I will not consent that this error, in which I delight, be wrested from me. But if it is true, as some insignificant philosophers maintain, that there is no soul, and that when dead I shall be deprived of all consciousness, then I shall not be afraid of dead philosophers laughing at my error." This is an elegant fortitude, but one that shows its painfully doubt-ridden infrastructure. Let Cato brag, and pose as the intrepid Roman senior citizen: he fools no one. For so long as those two "ifs" are there—"If I err . . ." and ". . . if it is true . . ."—ever so sharp, like the two fangs of soul-rending dubiety, we know that the heart cannot be at peace.

Neither science, nor religion, nor philosophy suffices to extricate us from the pangs of progressive bodily ruin and the anxiety of approaching death. Still, some, like Aldous Huxley, maintain that "the last line of defense is love." And though it may sound like cant or triviality, it is yet the best shield that one can interpose between old age and despair. Lucky those who in old age have some one person to care for, who cares for them. It remains undeniable that hope arises from depth of feeling more often than from keenness of intellect. Thus, Huxley's insight remains valid, that only "those who have learned the infinitely difficult art of loving all their neighbors" stand forever unhurt by insentience and apathy. And we, in our turn, owe a greater debt of love to the old than a general sentiment of affection and solidarity. For love of neighbor seems utilitarian: it springs from the consciousness that a certain comradeship is necessary among those who share in a common task. Whether we are conscious of it or not, all our acts are part of a larger plan, and our lives are like the bricks or the marble slabs on the walls of a palace: some crafted to perfection and deposited with pride, others of slovenly workmanship and uncritically laid down. But the aged are those who preceded us in the cosmic endeavor, and who now, no longer able to stand shoulder-to-shoulder with us in the wearisome toil, rest a tired brow by the shade of the rising walls. Our lives remain stressful, fragmentary, changeable, and uncertain, but theirs are hallowed by the touch of time. Their existence has run full circle, and they now prepare themselves to enter into the abyss of what is no more. Our debt of love is accrued of gratitude and admiration. Let us not forget that if they were no freer from the vices of their age than we are from such as sully ours, at least they did their duty: they secured, preserved, and transmitted to us whatever truths, freedoms, and comforts we have to lighten our present burden. And if we are not blind with rancorous prejudice, we shall acknowledge that they also provided us with that unit of measure by which we can continue to identify all that is lasting and excellent. They may have made mistakes, from which we suffer. But in balance the old were honest in intent, constant in misfortune, undaunted by fate, and generous of splendid examples to inspire us in the continuance of the unfinished task. May it please God soon to avert the terrible ills that now afflict so many amongst them.

Sexual Undifferentiation

In the year of our Lord 1655 was born, in the small town of Pourdiac, near Toulouse, France, a girl by the name of Marguerite Malaure. The curious have remarked in her family name, Malaure, a likeness of sound with *malheur,* misfortune, thus intimating that an unfavorable constellation presided over the hour of her birth and augured the unhappiness that later befell her. Orphanhood was the first in the list of her afflictions, for soon after entering this world she was left destitute of that precious warmth and protection that the majority of us find in the love of our parents. The good priest of Pourdiac saw to her early rearing, though with less thoroughness than her natural father might have used in educating a child of his own. She was placed in the service of an important lady, and it was in this office that she became a young woman. Undistinguished by social rank, physical beauty or talent, she comported herself, nonetheless, with dignity joined to engaging simplicity. Her pleasing disposition earned her general esteem, and her conduct was never known to furnish an occasion for reproach. In 1686 she fell ill, and had to be transported, feverish and semiconscious, to the Hôtel-Dieu, the hospital in Toulouse.

It is from that year that the first revelation of her baleful destiny can be dated. The physician who examined her declared, with wild displays of emotion ill befitting his noble charge, that he had never before encountered anything like Marguerite's sexual anatomy. She was endowed, he insisted, simultaneously with male and female procreative organs. She was male and female, instead of either one or the other, like the rest of us. More properly speaking, she was neither. To his astonished listeners, who were yet more ignorant than the medico and who stared at him as if uncertain that they had heard correctly, he addressed a pedantic speech sprinkled with heavy dashes of incorrect Latin at all the proper junctures. No one understood the learned explanation of Marguerite's freak-ish constitution, but all gave their hearty assent to the conclu-sion: Marguerite was not a she, but a he. On the authority of Aesculapius, Hippocrates, Galen, and other distinguished figures of medical science quoted by the doctor, a person must belong to one sex only, and if the marks of both happen to concur in the same individual, the one that is dominant must be chosen; the second one can be completely disregarded. Now, in Marguerite, maleness dominated, according to the doctor's report. (What the criteria for dominance were was not defined, but it suffices to recollect that, where dominance is concerned, maleness rarely came out the loser in the past.) Therefore, maleness was her manifest destiny. Therefore, for the previous thirty-one years of her life, she (or rather, he) had made a travesty of nature's decrees.

On the weight of this expert's deposition, the authorities de-manded that she take men's clothes and behave, thenceforth, in the ways most conformable to her newly acquired gender. This Marguerite found it impossible to do. Not only was she convinced that the doctor's ignorance did violence to her na-ture, but she had to face public scandal and harassment. An unhealthy collective curiosity was whetted that sought satisfac-tion at the expense of her honor and her modesty. The towns-men clamored for public exhibition of the subject of contention. She was accosted on the streets, insulted, humiliated by catcalls, and even soberly admonished by a priest to unveil what modesty enjoins to conceal, in the interest, he said, of the common weal and the advancement of science. Rather than waiting for the time when might would force what sophistry could not inveigle, Marguerite decided to leave town.

She took up residence in Bordeaux, where for a few years her life coursed unperturbed. But it was appointed that she would not enjoy a placid life. In 1691 a fellow Toulousian, passing through Bordeaux, recognized her and denounced her to the authorities. On July 21, 1691, an order of arrest was issued against her. There was a trial, and the verdict was that "her legal name shall be Arnaud de Malaure; she shall use men's clothes; and shall be forbidden, on pain of the whip, to dress like a woman." She was set free, but her future was severely compromised. Her education was limited, her skills rudimentary, and her very livelihood dependent upon being employed as a maid, a job from which she was now disbarred, on account of the official injunction. Desperate, she wandered from town to town, but her notoriety always preceded her; everywhere she was looked upon as a kind of monster, and survived only through the charity of the tolerant few.

Harassed, persecuted, ostracized, and hungry, she resolved to go to Paris in search of a remedy for her plight. Here, she was seen by a renowned physician, Doctor Helvétius, who sought the assistance of a surgeon, Doctor Saviard. Had surgery attained a state of development sufficient to warrant reasonable hopes of success, a corrective operation might have been attempted. But in those times surgical interventions designed to correct malformations, even those less complex than Marguerite's, were sure to provoke disasters greater than the ills they intended to correct. Prudence prevailed, and Helvétius, Saviard, and others, after careful consideration of the puzzling anatomical details, concluded that Marguerite was, indeed, a woman, and that she was not in need of the benefits of surgery. It remained, then, to reverse the sentence formerly passed by the courts of Toulouse. Marguerite's sorry lot, already pitiable on account of poverty, unemployment, suspicion, and societal rebuke, was compounded by the necessity to struggle against an archaic and difficult bureaucracy. She managed, in spite of all, to address a supplication to the king, who appointed a commission to look into the matter. In the end, experts were charged with the duty to reexamine the patient. This time judgment went for womanhood, but years of her life had been consumed in an arduous and painful struggle. Little is known about the details of her private life. History consigns to us only the fact that a trivial accident of birth, by producing a minor deviation in the somatic structure of a citizen of one of the most advanced countries of Europe, condemned the sufferer to a life of dejection and misery. Those who can read behind the factual descriptions of historical narrative will not fail to see, in addition, the courage, the dignity, and the admirable resiliency of a human being whose sole recompense for a life of appalling harshness was the right of wearing skirts, of bearing the name Marguerite, and of comporting herself, in public, like the woman she always thought she was.

History also shows that events of this kind were not precluded by the advent of an age that professed to be guided by the opinions of savants and philosophers. In effect, the age that we call the Enlightenment viewed developmental aberrations in the sexual sphere through less than enlightened glasses. The following example will suffice to illustrate these statements.

In 1732, Mr. Jean-Baptiste Grandjean and his wife, Claudine, became the proud parents of a newborn girl, whom they named Anne. Her childhood years went untroubled under the watchful vigilance of the convent sisters, to whom was entrusted the impartment of the early rudiments of learning and the sowing of the first seeds of the Christian faith in Anne's young mind. Nothing portended the astounding developments that were to come, until the girl entered puberty.

With the onset of adolescence, a tempestuous and heretofore unsuspected disorder made itself felt. At the age at which normal children experience the first tugs of sexual attraction to individuals of the opposite sex, or as was said at the time, "the birth of passions," Anne realized that nature had contrived to play her a distressing trick. Much to her confusion and alarm, all her troubling bestirrings were provoked by the proximity of girls, whereas in the presence of boys—precisely opposite to everyone's expectations—her inner self remained cold and impassive. This was, to the least perceptive, justifiable cause for alarm. She sought advice from her parents. They confirmed that, in addition to the described troubling preferences of Anne's soul, there were signs of bodily development that have always been regarded as sure signs of masculinity. The distressed family went to the confessor. This one, on grounds theological rather than scientific, resolved that Anne could not continue living under the guise of a girl, lest the occasions of sin be fostered in a most un-Christian way. For once, learned advice found a willing recipient. Anne desired nothing so much as to avail herself, or himself, of those natural utensils that nature had so surprisingly bestowed, and to do so under her current identity would be tantamount, said the confessor, to nothing less than abomination. Anne ceased to be Anne and took the name of her father, Jean-Baptiste. And with the change of name came not a change of heart (for the latter was already fixed in its natural preferences), but a change of attire, of comportment, and of public display. Masculinity was taken up with such alacrity that in a short time Jean-Baptiste's transmutation spanned the complete circle, from shy girl raised by the sisters, to lady-killer about town. Soon he was having a torrid affair with a Mademoiselle Legrand, and later, following the rupture of this dalliance, he became the lover of an experienced woman named Françoise Lambert. This time the union was more durable. Came the official engagement, the reading of the banns, and the celebration of matrimony on the 24th of June, 1761.

All was going well for Jean-Baptiste. Not only had he stumbled, as if by accident, on conjugal bliss, but his official status was confirmed. In effect, upon his decision to set up house in Chambéry, his father agreed to release to him a part of his inheritance. To do this, it was necessary to produce his birth certificate. The official in charge of legalizing the transaction read the official document, looked at the concerned parties with a glance of infinite bureaucratic apathy behind thick spectacles astride his nose, and, without further ado, scratched out the name Anne and wrote in its place Jean-Baptiste. Jean-Baptiste became a certified male.

It is not in vain that a philosopher once said that no man can declare himself happy until he is on his deathbed. Before that time the statement is always premature, for we do not know what new turn awaits us. This is well instanced by the life course of Jean-Baptiste. The couple had moved to Lyon, and lived happily, when Miss Legrand, Jean-Baptiste's former mistress, appeared before them. Hell hath no fury like a woman's spite. The mere spectacle of conjugal harmony was enough to spur her rancor. She managed to tell Mrs. Grandjean that Jean-Baptiste was less than a man, and that she pitied her for being legally and lastingly joined to a hermaphrodite. And she spiced her venomous sentences with all manner of intimate details, leaving it understood that she had full knowledge of these peculiarities by virtue of her former association with Jean-Baptiste.

Mrs. Grandjean was deeply troubled. Her experience in sexual matters had already taught her that, quantitatively speaking, her husband scored below average. On the other hand, nature admits of great variability within normalcy, and this happens, it is no secret, without detriment to quality. But presently, whatever doubts or reservations she may have had became sharply focused as a result of the unkind propositions slipped into her ear by the wretched intriguer. She suffered from the fact that there had been no children in her marriage; and in the midst of her present distress this frustration was sharply exacerbated. She opted to open her heart to her confessor, who became scandalized; inured to hear of the ills of this world, the priest found this complication unprecedented. His first disposition was to forbid Mrs. Grandjean all intimate commerce with her husband. For so long as a clear definition of gender was not available, all manner of intimacy was potentially sinful. This risk could not be run; it was better to remove all occasions to serve the devil. The reasoning of the theologian may have been flawless, but an age increasingly disrespectful of religious beliefs—and which had just produced a Voltaire—could not have failed to find it impugnable. Thus, in the wake of the public scandal produced by the *affaire Grandjean,* cynics were heard to say that it was strange that one confessor had advised Jean-Baptiste to do everything he could to affirm his maleness, while another confessor, drawing inspiration from the same faith, advised the wife to do all she could to deny what the husband had affirmed!

Jean-Baptiste, it goes without saying, was utterly confused and dejected. His wife's restlessness he found unjustified. How could he be expected to share her doubts? In the first place, he had lived with her for several years, having exerted all a husband's rights and duties without difficulty. Secondly, he knew full well that his ability to function in this department did not hang from a tenuous thread held by a single partner. To this Miss Legrand, the cause of his present worries, could well attest. Still more, his premarital activities further strengthened his confidence in the integrity of his manhood. Sexual potency in the male, though fragile and easily undone, will not come apart simply by the effect of ill-intentioned sayings spread around by a spiteful woman. Accordingly, Jean-Baptiste was not discouraged. He tried to dissuade his wife from her erroneous ideas, and even proposed to defer to higher arbitration. They could solicit, he said, the ruling of a high and respected prelate. He would willingly submit to the better judgment of a venerable mind that the troubled couple would agree in finding trustworthy.

A peaceful end to their worries did not come about. Before they could hear the words of comfort, they heard the bailiff knocking imperiously at their door. The secret of Jean-Baptiste's corporeal ambiguity had reached the office of the public prosecutor. Nor was it difficult to guess how this had happened.

All was due to Miss Legrand's solicitousness, and she was careful to couch her statements in words that showed Jean-Baptiste not as a victim of nature's inconsistency, but as a culpable agent acting deliberately to mock the laws of men. And so, we find Jean-Baptiste thrown into a dungeon, ball and chain to his ankles, with nothing but a heap of straw on which to rest his tired bones—fitting decor created by an era which was of a mind to build Bastilles. The charge leveled against him was no laughing matter: he was accused of willful profanation of the holy sacrament of matrimony, and wanton violation of the civil code. The punishment for these offences was severe. In previous times, it consisted of public dismemberment after torture with red-hot pincers. The growth of civilization had mollified these barbarous penalties. A generation before, the punishment was changed to death by hanging, removing all the gory prologue that had once thrilled the crowds. At the time of Jean-Baptiste's imprisonment, greater leniency had been introduced, but there was still good reason to be afraid: he faced the possibility of public whipping, a period of hard labor, and perpetual exile. In great haste, he interposed an appeal. His lawyers demanded expert testimony. They sought to prove, first, that the sex of their client was indeterminate or ambiguous; secondly, that the accusation of willful profanation of the holiness of matrimony was untenable. The first proof once accepted by the judges, the second argument would follow logically.

The royal physicians appointed as expert witnesses gave a lengthy deposition. The part dealing with the external physical examination of the accused contains the following description:

> In his external constitution the accused manifested a curious admixture of the two sexes in the same state of imperfection. He is beardless, but his legs are hairy, as are other parts of his body which generally are glabrous in women. He has more chest development than is commonly seen in men, but the breasts are not as delicate nor as sensitive to blows as they are in women. [This statement makes the modern reader shudder: were blows an integral part of the physical examination geared to establish the cor-

rect sexual identity of a patient?] His nipples, if one attends only
to their size, may be said to belong to the female sex, yet they do
not arise from the center of a dark red circle, as they do in women.
As for his voice, true it is that it corresponds neither to a man nor
to a woman; it is rather that of an adolescent boy, which lapses
now into acuteness, now into gravity of pitch, depending on the
capricious and unstable motions of the voice box.

From this report, the judges concluded that Jean-Baptiste
was, in fact, the victim of a developmental aberration that con-
ferred on him ambiguous genitalia. It yet remained to his law-
yer, Vermeil, to make use of all the oratorical strength and legal
expertise of which he was capable, if the announced punish-
ments were to be spared his client. In his moving address,
Vermeil developed the thesis that Jean-Baptiste could not have
acted maliciously to desecrate the holy vows of matrimony.
Profanation is possible, he said, only on condition that certain
well-defined circumstances prevail. In one case, the agent acts
under constraint, or somehow deprived of free will. This was
not applicable, since his client's marriage had been contracted
by the free and unimpeded choice of both spouses. In a second
set of circumstances, the conditions for abuse (of the holiness of
marriage) are met when one of the contractants knows himself,
or herself, incapable of discharging the prescribed duties and
obligations. In what concerns the sexual sphere, as contested,
the intent to deceive could not rightfully be charged to Jean-
Baptiste, who had actually cohabited with his bride before the
marriage ceremony. Lastly, one may be free and physically
capable, but make the wrong use of this capacity. Here again,
Vermeil's client was beyond reproach, as it was never alleged
that he consistently indulged in perverted or unnatural practices. Vermeil's pleading had the strength to convince the Par-
liament of Paris, which reversed the cruel decree issued by the
authorities of Grenoble. Jean-Baptiste was considered to be a
poor and ignorant fellow, whose acts were prompted by the
urgings of his abnormal nature unassisted by any restraint from
his natural limited understanding. Nevertheless, his good faith

was not in doubt. He recovered his freedom, but not the placid tenor of his former life. His marriage was declared null and void, and by a decree promulgated on the January 10, 1763, he was forbidden ever to marry again.[1]

What these stories show is that, of all our features, those that confer sexual identity most profoundly affect our lives. For who will deny that our vicissitudes in the world are linked to the simple and undeniable fact of being a man or a woman? Sex is, as some hotly contend, destiny. But why this must be so no one can explain. We are ready to accept sexual differentiation as a fundamental phenomenon of life; after all, the natural world is teeming with living beings to which different and complementary functions are assigned in procreation. But why sexual differentiation should also call for what biologists term "dimorphism"—that is, conspicuous physical differences between the sexes—is not immediately obvious. Nature seems not to enforce dimorphism in all its creatures: green algae *(Chlamydomonas)*, the sea urchin, or the sea star (echinoderms) are functionally split into males and females, but the respective appearances hardly differ from each other. And it is not the size, nor the simplicity of organization of a living being that matters. *Rotifera* is among the smallest metazoans known, yet males sharply differ from females: they are much smaller, and lack certain organs that females ostentatiously display. In contrast, snakes commonly show an almost identical appearance regardless of their sex; a small difference in the tapering of the tail, abrupt in females, gradual in males, is all that distinguishes the sexes. As to the dimorphism of our own species, it certainly does not belong with nature's flashiest. Ours are not the branched antlers of deer, nor the marked size disparities of oysters, nor yet the vivid, spectacular plumage of some birds. What passes in society for the decisive point of reference, or as the French colloquially put it, *"la différence,"* is the morphology of the external genital organs. Society has chosen to place here the focus of an exaggerated, hyperacute, and neurotic attention. Nevertheless, we cannot say that this is nature's most consummate product, nor the most boldly or trenchantly executed. For the external organs of human sexuality, those by which our fate is cast, are but a superficial layer, and the flimsiest, of a delicate series of formative processes that biology curiously disposes in a kind of onion-skinned arrangement.

At its central core, sex is said to be "genetic," since it is determined at conception. If the maternal egg cell, which carries one X chromosome, chances to be fertilized by a sperm cell carrying a similar X chromosome, a female will be engendered; if by a sperm cell carrying a Y chromosome, the conceptus will be male. Thus, this first difference is one felt to the most recondite part of our physical being, since all cells, without exception, contain a pair of like chromosomes in females (XX), whereas in the male the chromosomal constitution is dissimilar (XY). Here is an inflexible segregation that leaves no room for egalitarian claims, and peremptorily declares: Male and female are *not* created equal. However, genetic sex is only the first coiling; there are still myriad eventualities to be sorted out before sex organs are fashioned. The fertilized egg cell divides and gives rise to a tadpole-like creature that recapitulates, in a marvelously compressed time scale, I know not what primordial ancestors. By progressive transformations, the tadpole-like creature acquires the human shape, but not the sex. At about eleven weeks of gestation it looks like a miniature human being. All its major organs are formed, at least in basic outline, except those to which generation is entrusted. Seen from outside, the genital area of the embryo shows a diminutive phallus *(genital tubercle)*, identical in both sexes. The first of many incongruities of sex is thus made apparent. The conceptus is now made up of millions of parts—cells—all of which, individually, belong to one or the other sex, but the whole is nonsexed. Although dissection shows that sexual glands are found deep inside the embryo's flanks—"loins" is the accurate scriptural term for the anatomic substratum of sex—at this time they contain neither male sperm cells nor female egg cells. The early fathers of the Church pondered the biblical passage that says that man was created in God's image and semblance. Because it could not be supposed, without blasphemy, that God is sexed, some concluded that the first race of men must have been asexual, or hermaphroditic. In a sense, they did not err: in our earliest beginnings we belong to a sexually undifferentiated, bipotential race.

At about eleven weeks of gestation, sexual differentiation starts. As often happens, biology describes the "hows" in exquisite detail, but the "whys" are not always answerable. The Y chromosome, it is hypothesized, directs subsequent development toward maleness; without it, the male condition is impossible. It is by virtue of the information contained in the Y chromosome that the indifferent gonad becomes a testicle. And this is not all: once formed, this gland contributes, in its turn, to orchestrate the rising symphony of maleness. Its hormones abet the resorption or disappearance of those internal structures that *might* have given rise to a female genital system, and strengthen those that form adjuncts to the male apparatus. The prebirth formative process is then completed. The new being has reached the stage at which it is to be launched into the world. The obstetrician may now cast a cursory glance at this most external layer of the concentric formative coiling (while busy attending the dramatic proceedings of birth), and hurriedly exclaim: "It's a boy!" However, differentiation is not over. More layering is to take place at puberty, when all that is incidental or tangential to sex will receive the final touches. The male's voice deepens; his skin becomes hirsute. The female's breasts grow, her pelvis widens; and her bodily fat redistributes around the pelvic osseous enclosure with that fastidious precision that Marañón once compared to a careful padding, designed to shield from impact the precious object that will be housed therein.

It is hardly surprising, given the complex nature of the sequence, that mishaps occur. At conception, the chromosomes may be deficient (XO), excessive (XXY, or XYY), broken, unevenly distributed, or malfunctioning. The gonads may fail to form, or other aberrations may take place: a testicle on one side, an ovary on the other; ovary and testis fused into one gland (ovotestis) also occur, giving reality to the myth of Salmacis and Hermaphroditus, of which spoke the ancient poets. The bizarre stories can be read in the medical journals: A young man, athletic and vigorous, of normal sexual drive, is seen in the clinic because of a hernia that developed while weight-lifting. The surgeon discovers, inside the hernial sac, a perfectly formed uterus and Fallopian tubes, ignored relic of man's bipotential state that failed to regress despite apparent normalcy of all the attributes of the male sex. Conversely, a woman learns, after her entire childhood and part of her adult life had been spent in the attitudes, convictions, and beliefs that are proper to womanhood, that she is "really" a man: her cells possess the Y chromosome; perchance a male gonad is discovered in the abdomen, or in the inguinal canal.[2]

The troubling character of this pathology is owed to the last layer wrapped around the concentric biology of sex, and the most powerful: that of the mind's perception of sexual identity. For we are not distressed by the sexually ambiguous in quite the same way as by the sight of the lame, or the blind. It is not merely the spectacle of dysfunction or invalidity that troubles us. It is the perception of a travesty of values that we hold sacred, a bizarre foolery that mocks the emotions that poets have sung with their most exalted stanzas, and that threatens us all by detracting from the preservation of the race. Dysfunction is, nevertheless, a conspicuous handicap, for inasmuch as sexual coupling is a question of joinery, it remains governed by the same mechanisms that apply to mortises and tenons. The ancient Indian erotic treatises used quaint zoological metaphors to emphasize the need for correct anatomical coupling. Men's normal sexual organs corresponded to one of several precisely defined types: rabbit, deer, monkey, horse, and so on. And since this typology had its counterpart among women, the Indian sages insisted at great lengths on the necessity to join only those types that were compatible, such as woman-elephant with man-horse, placing no credence in the happiness of a couple whose sexual anatomy belonged to size-discrepant or mutually averse animal species. The male patient with disorders of sexual differentiation was said to fall entirely outside of this zoological typology, but in some cases his anatomy was judged compatible with women that the Indian *Sutras* analogized with the least sexually active of animal species. However, the sexually ambiguous were not always pariahs in the ancient creeds of India. In the time of the Moghul emperor Akbar thrived the sect of the *anubbashya-s,* in which men deliberately cultivated the feminine elements of mind and body. Their Lord was Krishna, represented as a male human figure. Believers aspired to union with the deity, and since mysticism runs close to eroticism (as the community of language reveals), their belief led to the conviction that the devout would be rewarded for their piety with a feminine body uniquely conformed for sexual pleasure. The *Rasa Panchadhyayi* promised the faithful extraordinary delights in the embrace of Krishna, skilled in all the practices of amatory technique. To my knowledge, this is the only mystic-philosophical system in which states of sexual ambiguity were admired and welcomed, as bringing votaries closer to a union with the divine master. Notions akin to this idea could have accounted for the fact, unearthed by students of the ancient subcontinent, that in remote historical times many men took the raiment of women, imitated their gestures, and willingly shared with them the life of the harem.[3]

In the West, glorification of sexual ambiguity was rarely observed, and generally issued from suspect motives. The court of Henry III of Valois probably came closest to granting official sanction to such deviancy. This strange monarch, last of the Valois dynasty, joined a keen intelligence to a bizarre, depressive personality; history has yet to pass a definitive judgment on this singular man. A great promoter of the humanities and the driving force behind the admirable Edict of Poitiers, he was nonetheless given to appear dressed like a woman when presiding over official ceremonies. Covered with cosmetics, glittering with jewelry, surrounded by dogs and parrots, this strange king shocked his subjects by his unorthodox behavior. Of his transvestite antics, Agrippa d'Aubigné wrote:

Si bien qu'en le voyant chacun était en peine
S'il voyait un roi-femme, ou bien un homme-reine.

Those who saw him could not tell what they had seen,
Had it been a woman-king, or perhaps a man-queen.

Because the transvestite monarch could be generous with his cronies, he was soon surrounded by sycophants ready to imitate his mannerisms. The famous "minions" were described by an outraged critic in a pamphlet suggestively entitled "The Hermaphrodites." In the satire, one of the minions states: "Why should one be condemned to be a man or a woman? It is so much better to be both at the same time, and thus to double one's pleasure. . . ." Clearly, the sixteenth century was not ready for Henry. Before he could manage to give governmental approval to hermaphroditism, the dagger of a fanatic regicide cut his life short, and with it ended what may have been the most bizarre chapter in the sexual mores of the ruling class.

Sexual undifferentiation is today regarded in a new light. Our age neither vituperates nor glorifies: it quantitates. We have thus learned that this pathology weighs more on the male than on the female side. For the male's functional adequacy is subject to morphologic unfolding. Because the male's copulatory role is an active one, nature must educe organs fit for this activity; the passive role of the female, in contrast, places no such demands for structural specialization. The female's outward genital organs differ but little from those of the embryo at the indifferent stage; the male's, if normal, progress to a phase of greater complexity. Yet, sophistication has a price in biology: simple functions are strong and abiding, and specialized ones are fragile and precariously maintained. Onrushes of blood, secretion of glands, cerebral concentration, well-timed nervous impulses and responses: a delicately balanced physiologic jugglery must be set in motion every time the male is to "perform." The female can, if she chooses, accomplish her assigned function, and even successfully conceive, with no need to polarize her entire physiology for the purpose. In a pornographic engraving of the school of Boucher, a courtesan suffers the forward charges of an undeceived customer while wistfully glancing at an open magazine. This intrinsic lability haunts the male's subconscious, and explains his exaggerated responses. Anxiety over his comparative inferiority and thinly propped functional ability leads him to react like the avaricious man that fears for his fortune. Maleness must be secure from all threats and perpetually guarded. A sort of jealousy, then, is the foundation of *machismo;* fear of the ever-threatening collapse of a function known to be feebly sustained. Accordingly, all imaginable reinforcement must be summoned. It is not enough to abhor all mannerism, dress, gesture, or attitude that directly betoken detriment to maleness; no hint that might undermine the male's idea of his own virility can be tolerated. In Mexico, one of many societies in which *machismo* reigns supreme, an actor that years ago enjoyed immense popularity, Pedro Armendáriz, refused to wear short-sleeved shirts on the grounds that such garments were unmanly. The famous film director Luis Buñuel tells us in his memoirs that he was forced to change the script of a murder scene in which the actor was stabbed in the back, dragged himself on the floor, dying, and asked of another actor to remove the knife from his back. The lines that Armendáriz was supposed to utter made reference to "this thing driven into me from behind." Notwithstanding the obvious dramatic context of the scene, the actor could not be persuaded to pronounce these words. Indistinctly he saw, as did Hamlet the ghost of his father, fogged but threatening, the terrifying specter of homosexuality, of maleness thwarted, diminished or vanquished.[4]

It is no coincidence that the same societies that have most zealously endorsed the affirmation of manhood have also inflicted upon it the bloodiest, most pitiless mockery and vilification. In the early postwar years there appeared in Mexico City a mysterious personage known as Count Balmori. Presumably, he descended from an old European aristocratic lineage, and had chosen to settle in the New World out of disappointment and frustration with the senseless carnage that had decimated the old continent. Rumor had it that he was immensely rich, having succeeded in transferring the family fortune at the start of the hostilities. He was said to possess a large estate in Spain, whose loss he had once feared, but which was now secure after the victory of the pro-monarchical forces of General Franco. He was also reputed to own copper mines in Chile, and a considerable share of stock in a San Francisco-based shipping company.

The Creole upper crust opened their doors to the exile, just for swank; and the ladies, always sensitive to the romantic spectacle of the man of distinction prey to homelessness and disillusion (a little à la Lord Byron), seemed less than eager to bolster the doors of their hearts in the presence of the blue-blooded gentleman. His perfect Castilian accent, the immaculate gloss of his well-starched collars, a somewhat old-fashioned cape that covered his shoulders, and a silver-headed ebony cane that twirled nonchalantly at the tip of his fingers: all the personal appurtenances and manners of the man enhanced his aura of distinction and polish.

There were, however, two things wrong with the lordly gentleman: he was neither titled, nor a man. As it became known later, Count Balmori was nothing but a terribly unkind hoax. A group of pranksters, annoyed by the ungenerous and obtuse ways of the many parvenus who in post-revolutionary Mexico oppressed the people (having forgotten their own origins), decided to play a humiliating turn on these nouveaux riches. A middle-aged woman was recruited to impersonate the fictitious count, and she displayed such a gift for acting, became so utterly immersed in her assigned role, that the deception was perfect. The results vastly exceeded the expectations of the japers. Buffoonery grew beyond the bounds of pure farce, and into the grounds of the absurd, the equivocal, and the dangerous. It became something that was not simply funny, and came very close to tragedy. Women became genuinely infatuated with the fake Count; jealousies festered; death threats were made; ugly scenes exploded. And every time, just inches away from bloodshed, Balmori would enact a grandiose finale. In the presence of expectant witnesses carefully arrayed by her cohorts, the actress would shed all her Balmorian paraphernalia: off with the wig, loosening a female head of hair; down with the fake mustache, revealing a hairless upper lip; away with the old-fashioned cape, disclosing a feminine bodily conformation. In place of the mysterious nobleman—for whose sake the guileless victims had compromised their social position, exposed themselves to public obloquy, or challenged the values dearest to conventional morality—there stood a rather plain-looking woman, one of the many undistinguished members of the mestizo proletariat that the rich daily ignored with arrogant disdain. This sort of humiliation, as we may suppose, coursed in silence. The victims were never keen to lend voice to their indignation, which would only have widened the reach of their shame. It was thus possible for the pranksters to restart a new cycle. And such is the uncharitableness that may hatch in the human heart, that not uncommonly the victims, now privy to the secret, relished the preparation of the trap for the next victim.

The story of the infamous Balmori is no fiction; the authenticity of its episodes is backed by relatively fresh testimony. A skillful writer might one day exploit the rich color and psychologic intricacy of the Balmori scandals. But there is no dearth of this kind of material, however outlandish it might seem at first sight.[5] Many are the examples of women who have passed for men, and vice versa. Catalina de Erauso, in the sixteenth century, pushed male impersonation to the extreme. She joined the army and distinguished herself in military actions. Described by a biographer as "the wildest and most turbulent of all female transvestites in history," she killed her own brother, who, unaware of her identity, thought that she was a rival with designs on his mistress. Then, there was Maximiliana von Leihorst (died August 29, 1748), who renounced her sex at fourteen, also joined the army, participated in the Turkish campaign, and would have attained the highest military honors but for the sad circumstance that she developed cancer of the breast, and could no longer conceal her true identity. She died at the age of forty-four years. In industrial England there was the notorious case of James Allen, who was actually a woman, but who thought herself a man with such strong conviction that on December 13, 1807, she married an Abigail Naylor. The femaleness of James Allen came to public notice only when she died in consequence of a job-related accident and the body was examined by the coroner. Sensational journalism was not tardy in exploiting this oddity. It was then hinted that the surviving wife was actually a man, "Naylor," just as the deceased husband had actually been a woman. When, on January 17, 1829, the body was deposited in a vault at St. John's Bermondsey ("precautions being taken to prevent the malign activities of the resurrection men," says the biographer), a huge crowd gathered that vented the most reprehensible prejudice by insulting the poor widow. They shouted at her when she ventured out. Insolent Peeping Toms roamed about her house, and looked through windows, holes, cracks in the walls or doors, hoping to confirm by direct inspection what the rumors were saying. It was claimed that the Good Samaritan Society refused to extend its charity to the suspect widow, and although this was probably an exaggeration, there is little question that the most vexatious pressure must have been experienced by Abigail, because she decided to look for a magistrate in whose presence she signed an affidavit that, she hoped, would clear her name. In it she states, after the customary legal terminology identifying the deposer as Abigail Allen of No. 32 East Lane, Rotherhithe, that she was "entirely ignorant of the fact of the said James Allen being a female, until that circumstance was communicated to me by the woman who undressed the body after death." We know no more of the unfortunate widow(er), but the line of impersonations continues unbroken to our day. In 1943 a Chicago child photographer, who had previously been a truck driver, a gang boss, and the owner of a construction company, was exposed as being "in reality" (perhaps we should say, in addition) a woman. She had married the daughter of an Akron physician, and although the wife became aware of the sex of her spouse, she saw no reason to dissolve the marriage. Rather, she wished to cement their union further, with a child. The couple decided to illegally acquire one, which they were to buy, while pretending that it was naturally begotten. Their scheme was ruined when the wife's father became suspicious at not being permitted to examine his own daughter, notwithstanding his medical qualifications.

One finds with equal ease, throughout the world, examples of two men living in wedded bliss and contriving to deceive society in order to avoid its harsh reproof. As recently as November, 1984, the Taiwan newspapers disclosed the story of a policeman who had managed to marry, with all the rites and ceremonies that attend betrothals in the Orient, another man disguised as a woman, and who had previously married a woman (a real one, the previous one, the newspapers implied). I will dispense with the details of the case, which in a conservative society, such as Taiwan's, where traditional roles are meticulously respected and reinforced by a strict government, was bound to cause a sonorous scandal, from which the tabloids abundantly benefited. And yet, the Orient has ancient traditions linked to sexual undifferentiation. The ancient Kabuki theater of Japan cultivates, as is well known, the art of female impersonation by male actors. Something of the sort occurs in China, at least in the Peking Opera plays. Japanese connoisseurs insist that no woman could possibly represent the female roles so movingly. For it is not the realistic rendering of femininity that matters. This art aims at extracting a distillate, an essence, the idea of femininity in general, rather than a portrait of a particular woman. Only the male actors, the *onnagata,* can succeed in this task. An actress, by virtue of being a real woman, cannot help but carry with her the concrete portrait. But whereas women can never set themselves at sufficient distance from femininity to capture its vast and ethereal outlines, the *onnagata* can do so. It is an art that requires maturity and experience. A few years ago, a famous male actor, already in his seventies, acted in a play in which he had the role of the wife of a young warrior. Audiences were thrilled by his exquisite portrayal, while the actor with the role of husband in the play (in real life the older actor's son) moved around the stage clumsily and was denied the ovations lavished on his partner. Nor is it to be assumed that all this is restricted to the "classic" Japanese stage. The tendencies in which this tradition is rooted may show in popular, and sometimes vulgar, expressions of society. Kitsch is not alien to the Japanese. A people who balk not at adorning the streets with vases displaying plastic flowers, or playing electronic recordings of birds' warblings in department stores, could not be expected to cavil at artificiality in the spontaneous expressions of so-called pop art. Thus, in a Tokyo nightclub, the well-known female impersonator Miwa Akihiro entertains his audiences under a crystal chandelier, amidst statues of nude young boys and onyx vases displaying carefully arranged peacock feathers. An observer noted that, as the would-be woman singer intones her cheaply sentimental ballads, it is not unusual to witness burning tears roll down the cheeks of the male customers. Some of these may be sinister-looking types, possibly hardened criminals in their regular life, yet at the end of the performance they are heard to say in a voice trembling with emotion: "Madame never looked more beautiful than tonight!"[6]

Such is the baffling picture of sexual differentiation and undifferentiation. Here is yet one more mirror held up to the grandeur and misery of the body. It seems that our species was meant to be composed of individual beings exquisitely complementary to each other. Wherefore this sequential coiling, this concentric series of transformations, this portentous alchemy from which nature obtains the body in one of the two modes of its grandeur: male or female. Why, then, the last coiling, that of the mind, by which grandeur may turn to misery? For the mind, with Olympian stubbornness, may choose to deny the dumb striving of nature. The transvestite, conscious of belonging to one sex, derives vicarious pleasure from indulging in the external habits of its opposite. The homosexual yearns to become what he, or she, is not. The transsexual, that tragic entity, behaves "as if he were" what he plainly is not. And outside the circle of the tragic all move in confusion: one, the male supremacist; another one, the intransigent feminist; still another one, the pontificator or dogmatizer. Each vehemently thinks to hold the keys of femininity and masculinity, when, in fact, they have but confused, notional concepts. Their theory is reduced to the facile assumption that "boys will be boys and girls will be girls," for most live with the fixed delusion that there are two sexes, without gradations. But research increasingly makes plain that sex is a continuum, whose degrees and dimensions are just beginning to be understood. So that the study of intersexed persons has momentous importance; it is not simply the idle preoccupation of specialists with a bent for the odd. Nor is the role of those unfortunate persons simply to frazzle us at a circus side show. Understanding of sexual differentiation has become the sole avenue for cognition of the forms of human existence, which up to now has been dependent on our weak perceptions. Descartes, that French gentleman who taught the world the road to certainty, came up with a quaint allegory: We look through the window at the street below, and persuade ourselves that we see John and Mary—the rich subjectivity, the intricate texture of two human beings. But what we see is *"chapeaux et manteaux, rien de plus."* (Hats and coats, nothing else.) So it is with the sexes. We dress the thin sense-data with the rich garments of stereotype; we believe we see psychological attributes, expected behavior, assigned roles, position in society. But all we see is certain somatic features, perhaps certain genital anatomical configurations. Hats and coats, nothing else.

Mors Repentina:
An Essay on Three Forms of Sudden Death

BY LIGHTNING

Dr. Milton Helpern, in his capacity as Chief Medical Examiner of the city of New York, had ultimate responsibility for that ineffable task that consists in stamping the passport of those who unexpectedly embark for the beyond. For this passport, better known hereunder as the "death certificate," must be duly stamped; it must bear one of the three seals available for unnatural death: suicide, homicide, or accident—the mark of dishonor, pity, or indifference impressed upon it by the living. This task is not easy. As may well be supposed, in a place like New York City the manner of departure admits of infinite variations, and a correspondingly infinite number of possibilities must be reduced to one of three labels. To investigate the details of such abscondings is the chief function of the Chief Medical Examiner. Considering the limitations inherent in the retrospective methods used, this function is discharged admirably well. An example from Helpern's experience will amply illustrate these statements.

The remains of several adult men found in the underground transport system labyrinths were brought to the city morgue, at various times, for ascertainment of the mechanism of death.

The deceased were homeless derelicts known to the local police for vagrancy. Because the bodies were found on, or near, the tracks, badly mangled by a passing train, suicide or homicide seemed plausible hypotheses. The harrowing cast of life of the homeless in New York City readily makes suicide a possibility; defenselessness, a patent feature of this life, raises the likelihood of homicide: those familiar with this life know of the risk that the destitute daily run, of falling victim to the brutish sadism of other outcasts, more vigorous than the slain. But accident? Not likely, especially for those who moved in the passages of the subway system with the self-confidence and familiarity of men comporting themselves in their true and fixed domicile. Nevertheless, one anatomical finding, common to all the victims, came to clarify the mechanism, not to say the cause, of their demise: the penis of each one was utterly carbonized.

Their last moments could therefore be reconstructed. They had sought their nightly shelter in the labyrinths of the subway. They had come wearing their ill-fitting clothes, the neck of a bottle of hard liquor protruding from the rear pocket of the baggy trousers or the side pocket of the threadbare overcoat, three sizes too big. While above ground, they had resorted to frequent sips from their bottles to protect themselves from the cold; underground, they kept to the same expedient for reasons they had forgotten, or, at any rate, in order to forget that reasons were needed to justify this indulgence. What followed should be plain. It is a well-known fact—for which it is unnecessary to invoke scientific principles of physiology—that frequent libation and a cold ambient temperature promptly stimulate the urinary function. With their bladders filled to capacity, they had looked for a secluded turn of the subway passages to relieve themselves of the excess fluid. At a prudent distance, but perhaps from the edge of the platform when no passengers were around, they had released a stream of urine, which formed a continuous arched jet between their bladders and the train tracks. And as soon as the stream touched the tracks, the thousands upon thousands of volts of electricity needed to move

New Yorkers around, conveniently harnessed in the tracks, found an alternate route in the salt-rich fluid, and flowed in a fraction of a second into the body of the unwary vagrants.

Diagnosis: struck by lightning, underground.

Aboveground, death by lightning is known as the epitome of sudden death, and one appropriately decked in full dramatic regalia. The clouds part, and from heaven descends this flashing, stentorian, curiously stepped sickle that mows at random. And what further increases its terror, it makes our distress prescient: we know that an explosion is about to occur, we clearly sense it in the agitation of the storm, but cannot guess precisely when. With loud explosions all around us we are left to wonder whether we are to be the next target. *Media vita in morte sumus,* in the midst of life we are in death: nothing brings home the truth of this obvious dictum better than to find oneself out of doors in a thunderstorm. The zigzagged, forked, and streaked lightning flashes are followed by incredibly loud peals, ominous rumbles, or frightening claps. No matter how absurd or inopportune, the old injunctions keep coming back to us: do not place your feet in the water, do not stand under a tree. For over four decades I have resided in large cities, where lightning is "triggered" from high towers by that ingenious device whose design has not been altered since it was invented by Mr. Franklin in 1752. Like most city dwellers, I do not place death by lightning high on the list of my most feared accidents. However, the childhood memory of an evening spent on horseback, on a rugged mountain, caught in a thunderstorm and hurrying to reach the nearest haven, stands indelible in my mind. More frightening than the peals and rolls of thunder, more disquieting than the flashes whose unseen leaders briefly illuminated the clouds before we were sunk again in darkness, was the perceived uneasiness in the voice of my generally self-possessed mother, who prayed: "Into thy hands do I entrust my soul, O Lord. . . ." For a while, my childishness harbored a shade of resentment against her, for having failed to measure up, on that occasion, to Marguerite of Austria, who took to composing verses for her own epitaph while on a tempest at sea, or to André Chénier, who walked, rhyming, to his decapitation.[1]

But for those exceptional circumstances, death by lightning loses its frightening mask. It seems remote and improbable, the sort of liability we can be complacent about. Nor is any amount of information about to change our smugness and unconcern. It is a scientifically demonstrated fact that about 40,000 thunderstorms shake the earth's atmosphere per year, discharging, on the average, 8,000,000 flashes of lightning, ten times more frequently over land than over water. But it is equally true that fewer than 100 persons die annually by such mechanism in the United States. Compared to the yearly carnage on the highways, lightning-associated mortality hardly deserves a fleeting thought from statisticians. Vulcan's forge atop Mount Etna was an awesome image to the ancients, who trembled before the unopposable fury of lightning. Yet, Vulcan's forge is to Detroit's assembly lines as the slingshot to the teleguided missile. City dwellers are not worried by lightning, and it would take no less than the full staging of a thunderstorm to distress them. In Herman Melville's short story "The Lightning-Rod Man," the salesman disposes of only a brief time favorable for business. He must wait for the skies to blacken, and the wind to hit the shutters, and the slanting rain to shake the sashes, before he chooses to appear to peddle his copper lightning-rod, at a dollar a foot. Were it not that such "special effects" punctuate his every argument, he would stand no chance of selling his wares. The storm dissipates, and the main strength of his salesmanship goes with it. The resistant buyer, resettling into self-assurance, can say: "In thunder as in sunshine I stand at ease in the hands of my God. False negotiator, away! See, the scroll of the storm is rolled back; the house is unharmed; and in the blue heavens I read in the rainbow that the Deity will not, of purpose, make war on man's earth."

Quite so. The Deity has, I suspect, much better means of attrition than thunderbolts. Lightning can scarcely be a divine weapon to make war on man's earth. Rather, it is His gentle reminder, made plain on selected occasions, as in those reported instances in which lightning has traversed an aircraft in flight without harm to its passengers. It is a fillip from the Almighty, translated into forest fires that amount to yearly losses of millions of dollars. It is a pat from on high, raining down on us in the form of 8,000,000 thunderbolts per year, of which only a few, now and then, have been known to knock down a cruising DC-10 with all its passengers, or to strike a golf player surprised by an unseasonable thunderstorm while wearing shoes with metal cleats on the soles.

As for those wretched tipplers who fell struck by lightning under the ground, they cannot be the targets of His wrath. I have seen others like them, oblivious or indifferent to warning signs, touched by high-tension wires and visited by comparable deaths—though I have not seen, it must be owned, the visitation gain entrance via the same anatomic route as in Helpern's cases. And what struck me the most was not the unusual nature of their end—those struck down in the subterranean labyrinths —but the reaction that it evoked in the living. I often sensed, even in those who did not admit it, a certain sanctimoniousness, a certain urge to remonstrate that all was as it should be, that death by electrocution was a means of divine reproof. The ancestral idea of a nether world where retributive justice is meted out as torment is too firmly entrenched in our subconscious. A subterranean accident can stir atavic images of fire emerging from the underworld, from hell, to strike at the unholy; more strongly than is commonly supposed, this idea is made to apply to fatal accidental electrocution on empty lots, in ill-guarded plants of the power company, and above all, to that strangest of all sudden deaths: death by lightning. However, before the Judeo-Christian code of guilt and expiation became thoroughly engraved in our minds, the Greeks believed that death by lightning made the victim godlike, raising him to everlasting glory. The flash that strikes down Semele, at one and the same time raises her to heaven; Heracles, for the same reason, vanishes from the pyre set on fire by Zeus's lightning. For the sacred fire of lightning was thought to possess a dual power: it was the tool of destruction, and the instrument of purification, for mortal man. When the bones of Lycurgus were transported back to Sparta for burial, writes Plutarch, lightning struck the grave in which they were placed. This, no doubt, was the gods' posthumous honor to the lawgiver; on the authority of Pliny (*Nat. Hist.* 7:152) we know that the same distinction went to Euthymos, when the statues of this Olympic champion at Locri and Olympia were struck by lightning. The Greeks believed that the body of a person struck by lightning was incorruptible; dogs and birds of prey dared not touch it, and it had to be buried at the same place where lightning had struck.

Dissectors: Careful, if you should encounter a victim of urban lightning. Approach those remains with more than the usual respect. You may have, without knowing it, the remnants of a hero at the tip of your scalpels. Remember, too, that the same death was reserved for Asclepios, the father of all physicians and the founder of Medicine,[2] who was struck down by the flash of Zeus and granted the constellation of Ophiucus for eternal dwelling. Who knows? Like Asclepios, those wretched boozers might have emerged as deities: *Aesculapius, ut in deum surgat, fulminatur.*

BY ASPHYXIATION

More than any other bodily function, respiration signifies life. It is the very first visible sign by which the newly born manifest their arrival into the world of the living. And the belief is widespread in primitive societies that the life-giving principle is a breath which enters man at his beginning and leaves him at his end, when in the act of "breathing his last" the activating vital principle quits the body through the mouth, to return to the airy environment whence it came. In the Upanishads, name, form, and action are presented as the trinity of the universe, but those three are reduced to one: *Atman,* understood as "breath," the Spirit of Life. In the Praśna Upanishad, when the sage is asked what are the powers that keep the union of a being, and "how many keep burning the lamps of life," the reply mentions at least three connected with respiration: space, air and voice. In the Judeo-Christian cosmogony, "the Lord God formed man out of the dust of the ground, and breathed into his nostrils the breath of life" (Gen. 2:7). The method has not changed when Ezekiel has a vision of dry bones restored to life (Ezek. 37:9): Ezekiel invokes the spirit from the four winds, so that, when it breathes from the four quadrants on the slain, an army of resuscitated men spring to their feet.

In the very act of our generation the agency of air has often been invoked. In the *Problemata Physica,* Aristotle linked air and sexual desire. In Problem XXX, I, the froth that forms on wine is adduced as proof that it has the quality of generating air, in contrast with oil, which forms no froth even when it is hot. Wine owes its aphrodisiac effect to this quality; for a man in his cups, says the philosopher, is often inclined to embrace and kiss even those who, when sober, would never elicit from him such outbursts. To the Stagirite the phenomenon of penile erection is only comprehensible if it is accepted that it is due to inflation by air, for no other mechanism is compatible with the rapidity of its onset. He maintained that an excess of "pneuma" determines the libido of melancholics (*De generatione animalum* 728, 9), whose airy surfeit shows itself in the inflated veins that course through their foreheads. And even prepubertal boys derive a pleasurable sensation from rubbing their genitals out of wantonness, "the manifest reason being that the air escapes through the passage through which the fluid flows later on." This rudimentary conception of physiology may make us smile, yet in it is the fundamental truth that life is drawn in, that its ingress is made by insufflation. Then it leaves us, the next moment, through what is aptly called "expiration." Inhale-exhale: these two brief movements condense and summarize our entire existence. Its brevity, its dumb momentum of automatic pumping in and puffing out, for no other reason than its deep and obscure striving, puts in our lips the lamentation of Job: "My days are swifter than a weaver's shuttle; they come to an end without hope. Remember that my life is like the wind . . ." (Job 7:6–7).

Our life is like the wind, transient and insubstantial. How else could it rest wholly on as thin a support as breath? Nothing tells more of the frailty of the human condition than its complete subordination to this airy influx. The infinitely complex series of physico-chemical phenomena that we call material life depends for its sustenance on a mere breeze, a thin current of air traveling in and out of our lungs. We sense here an incongruity. It seems as if our design had been made strangely vulnerable, not to say imperfect. For there is a weak link in the system: the windpipe. The function of the airway is delicately balanced, carefully monitored, but it narrows into a vulnerable strait, a treacherous pass. Unlike simple organisms, who "breathe" across their entire bodily surface, air must come to us swirling across this bottleneck. Hence, a minor swelling will make us wheeze, and a trivial object—an olive, a cherry, or a small pebble—may kill us. The fatal sequence is well known. The victim engages in the simple pleasure of eating. Minutes before, he enjoyed a hearty laugh upon the utterance of a joke, or a witticism from the guests at the table. Then, a small, thin, smooth or slick fragment of food inadvertently slips through and enters the pharynx, the threshold of the narrow pass. The victim senses the threat, and almost automatically makes a deep inhalation attempting to regain his breath. But these intense respiratory efforts are counterproductive: they widen the pharynx and the larynx, and the foreign object penetrates more deeply. Terror now seizes the victim, who clutches his throat and gesticulates, unable to speak. In seconds, air, space, and voice—the powers of life of which the Upanishads spoke—are instantaneously cut off from him. Panic strikes at his heart, and rarely spares the observers; it dilates his pupils and throws him into a pathetic, agitated despair. He turns bluish, and unless the occluding object is quickly expelled, he loses consciousness, and is dead within minutes.

In the medical literature this manner of death, "the café coronary," as it was styled by Haugen in 1963, loses none of its drama.[3] The victim is middle-aged, or elderly; the weapon, a fragment of filet mignon, a piece of broiled lobster, a morsel of bread, or sundry other foodstuffs. Regarded in this light, French fries look like veritable bullets, and as deadly. Bullets themselves, quietly, unheralded by explosions, have been known to wreak their lethal devastation by plugging the airway. Thus, in what is probably the first English-language account of this accident, Robert Hooke read to the members of the Royal Society of London, in 1677, a letter that detailed an instance of accidental occlusion of the airway by pistol shots. The patient, a Mr. Williamson, of Cornwall, had attempted "to cure himself of colic" by the then fashionable expedient of swallowing musket balls. On April 12, 1674, his faith in this treatment undaunted, he swallowed three pistol shots. One of these was said to be lodged in the trachea, and could not be expelled, despite his being suspended by the heels and made to inhale fumes of "Storax," "Benjamin," and other suitable preparations from the seventeenth-century pharmacopoeia.[4]

Our era has abandoned these therapies in favor of gaining a closer look at the suffocating threat. According to Mittelman and Wetli, the overall risk of sudden death from "café coronary" is 0.66 per 100,000 population.[5] It increases with age, so that for an individual seventy years of age or older, the figure rises to an alarming 14 per 100,000 population. The fact is, most lethal risks increase with age, for life must come to an end. And there are those who argue that a swift one that arrives amidst cheerful libation and conviviality, after a long life, is neither contemptible nor frightening, and may be sparing of a more hurtful finale. Perhaps. On the other hand, a child's choking on foodstuffs and foreign objects is a most grievous and sorrowful occurrence, and choking is the leading cause of accidental death in the home for children under one year of age. Of those below five years, at least as many die from asphyxiation as from accidental poisoning. The killers: candy, nuts, grapes, and a variety of dainties whose "index of lethality," if calculated by a researcher overpreoccupied with the meaninglessness of the universe, would surely be shown to be proportional to their ability to delight. One curious fact is worth noting: statistics reveal that more than forty percent of all deaths by suffocation in which the foodstuff is specified are due to hot dogs and candies.[6] Cooling of patriotic ardor notwithstanding, this quintessentially American invention, the hot dog—which every staid citizen, established proprietor, and chamber of commerce throughout the land wishes to see in the hands and mouths of all children at national festivities—turns out to be a potentially deadly tool. So risky, that it smacks of demoniac creation. For one may well imagine an intelligent evil spirit pondering over the design of the most appropriate instrument for accidental suffocation: considering the shape and dimensions of the oropharynx, and the mechanics of deglutition, the deadly object should have certain physical characteristics. Its shape should be cylindrical; its surface should be smooth, so as to glide almost imperceptibly; it should be compressible, but resilient; undigestible by oral secretions; soft, but not friable. . . . In one word: the hot dog.

"Our fight," the historian Herbert Butterfield pronounced, "is against some devilry that lies in the very process of things, against something that we might even call demoniac forces existing in the air." He was referring to destructiveness and irrationality in human action, as perceived through a detached contemplation of history. But the statement applies, literally, to death by suffocation. In Blankaart's seventeenth-century medical dictionary asphyxia was defined as a perceptible deficiency of the pulse (from *a* privative, and *sphyzo,* I jump).[7] The Oxford Dictionary of Etymology says: "stoppage of the pulse, (hence) suffocation." Thus, the idea of a lethal oppression, or compression, is there; a weighing-down upon the victim until the vital pulsation is no more. And the irrational (but surely no less respectable for that) idea that the efficient cause of this pressure lies with a demon springs to mind when one reflects upon the overwhelmingly absurd fact that human life, that precious product of eons of evolutionary striving and adaptation, can be stopped short by a piece of half-chewed Polish sausage.

There are also those who asphyxiate in their sleep. And although one thinks this exit quiet, it is, in many cases, a last struggle. Normal sleep should be accounted the sweetest of human experiences. For it is then that the soul gathers itself, said Plutarch, from its dispersed and diffused state throughout the senses, and becomes "like a slave who has escaped." And, turned pediatrician, Plutarch next informs us that infants never smile before the third week of life except in their sleep, because only then the soul succeeds in lifting itself above animal life, and thus enfranchised it evokes the delights enjoyed in a former existence. Contemporary medicine, however, has recently defined a condition in which the shocks and stresses of vigil do not relent, and the soul remains in bondage: the sleep apnea syndrome. Apnea is defined as an episode of cessation of air flow at the nose and mouth for at least ten seconds. Patients with this disorder experience at least thirty episodes of apnea each night; some suffer hundreds. Sleep loses its revitalizing powers, and slumber prolongs the miseries of wakefulness. Hence the fatigue, the sleepiness that plagues the victims during waking hours. Some report falling asleep at work; in one case, an episode of "micro-sleep" occurred while driving, and the sufferer narrowly escaped death when his car crashed against a barrier lowered in front of a passing train.[8]

Consider the recording that technology makes possible. Video tapes leave us with the impression that victims of sleep apnea struggle while asleep to remove an oppression. There are abnormal movements of the hands, and wider displacements of whole limbs, as if to cast off the offending pressure. There is inordinately loud snoring, then silences that extend for twenty or more seconds: the struggle is on, then interrupts itself, then renews itself once more. The X-rays show that the diaphragm stops its activity, as if the sleeper's thorax had been clamped into immobility by a great weight. But where is this weight? Above the patient, on top of his body; now on his chest, now on his throat. Polygraphic recordings show that the sufferer makes desperate attempts to draw in a whiff of air, but inspiration seems to be hampered by an obstacle. By a currently unknown mechanism, the walls of the pharynx in some patients suddenly collapse and occlude the airway. Death rarely follows in an otherwise healthy individual. But the effects of the loss of sleep and deficient respiration may be felt by even the strongest. The mind (or as Plutarch would say, the soul) suffers early: this fretful sleep is accompanied by frequent nightmares. For the restorative powers of sleep can only be subverted at great peril. The ancients believed that sleep puts us in a unique relation with the supernatural: revelations were apt to be received only during sleep and ecstatic states, which pry the receptive faculty loose from the body, leaving it free of all influences that trouble the purity of its perceptions. It is thus that sleep brings to the patient with sleep apnea frightful nightmares and, eventually, a distortion of the inner self: children may experience somnambulism, or regression to bedwetting after toilet training had been completed.

There is another graphic representation of sleep apnea, apart from that of polygraphic recordings. It is subjective and fanciful, but in a sense no less informative. I am speaking of *The Nightmare,* the famous oil on canvas of the Swiss painter John Henry Fuseli,[9] first shown at the Royal Academy of London in 1782, and today at the Detroit Institute of Art. The well-known composition depicts a young woman lying on a bed, clad in a virginal white sleeping gown, the upper third of her body hanging down from the edge of the bed toward the floor. She lies exanimate, in an attitude of utter defenselessness and abandon that could not fail to suggest to generations of critics the idea of sexual surrender (more so because, according to some art experts, the sexual overtones in the work of Fuseli are always far from veiled). Her fully extended left arm droops langorously, flaccidly, parallel to her cascading hair. The rendering of this posture strikingly achieves the effect of a loose body whose consciousness has been extinguished, or suspended. It is the posture of those prey to the nightmare. And to directly reinforce the certainty that the benumbed maiden is thus victimized, Fuseli placed, squatting on the lower chest of the girl, a horrifying monster or incubus. Its gleaming, reddish eyes stare fixedly at us from the center of the canvas. The incubus is the nightmare, "the being that lies on top of the sleeper." (Nightmare is still *incubo* in Italian, and we recognize in the verb "to incubate" [from the Latin *incubare*] the idea of "lying on top"). In popular traditions it appears as an animal, a small man, or an old woman, who exerts an oppression by sitting on the chest of the slumberer, thus suffocating—and sometimes copulating with—the latter. Adding to the theatricality of the scene, Fuseli painted a dark-red curtain as background, through which peers the head of a horse that looks at the girl and the incubus with wild, maddened, protruding eyes. The composition is completed by a small table at the foot of the bed, on which rest several objects, including a mirror. This one is so placed as to reflect on its surface the scene taking place in the bedroom, but, in fact, it reflects nothing. And one may well imagine here a parallel to the paradoxical findings of polygraphic recordings in patients with sleep apnea: the tracings point to a suffocating compression, but the incubus remains invisible. Modern medicine, however, does not disregard the incubus. It was an old superstition that to prevent the malicious attacks of incubi the potential victims ought to be prevented from lying flat on their backs, for this posture enhances their vulnerability. And so it is that I have heard resourceful pediatricians recommend to mothers of children with the sleep-apnea syndrome that they sew large buttons, or sewing-thimbles, to the back of the pajamas worn by the patients. This ingenuity aims at decreasing the time that the patient sleeps on his back, and thus the number of apneic attacks.

"Dream of a shadow is the life of man," wrote Pindar. Uncer-

tain, fragile, inconsistent, and brief, even for those to whom nature opened her generous prodigality. Fleeting and empty, like the froth formed at the surface of liquids that are shaken: buoyant one instant, vanished the next. And this simile became a proverb, whose inimitable conciseness reinforces the idea of brevity: *Homo, bulla* (Man is a bubble). One was choked by a grape, another succumbed to aspiration of the contents of his own stomach, still another was laid level in his sleep by the hand of an incubus. Such is the weakness of man, whose tempestuous undertakings agitate the whole planet, and who now, finding it too narrow a theater for his bold emprise, readies himself to venture forth into limitless space. Erasmus reviewed much of the plaintive literature on the brevity of life written in classical antiquity, and he regretted its concern with form over depth of feeling. As one who, by reason of his trade, has been often forced to look squarely at sudden death, I should like to paraphrase his melancholy apology and summation: "Many seem to enjoy such declamations and digressions. But in me, it was sheer pain, not the enticement of amenity, which induced these morbid reflections."

BY WE KNOW NOT WHAT

There are also those who die without our knowing why. There are military recruits who die in the prime of youth, during harmless drills, in the trenches. There are voodoo deaths in Haiti, and hex deaths in the United States. There is fatal arctic hysteria, *pibloktoq,* among Eskimos, and *susto* deaths (soul loss, magical fright) in Hispanic America. And there are deaths from sudden fright or violent emotions in all localities throughout the world. I have seen deaths without observable anatomical causes, and anatomic lesions whose relation with death is ambiguous or uninterpretable. And I have also seen—most puzzling phenomenon on which few seem to reflect—extensive lesions that caused the death of the one victim but spared another, though the lesions were seemingly identical in both. But there is one death that adds to puzzlement a persistent melancholy and a sense of helplessness. Such is the death of infants who die in their cribs.

The "sudden infant death syndrome" is perhaps the best known of sudden and unexpected forms of dying. It is not a culture-dependent folk illness; it is world-wide. The lay public is well aware of it. Yet one does not refer to it by its full and terrible name. Allusion is made by way of an acronym, SIDS; for the throttling demon is not to be named directly. It must be exorcised by cries with an esoteric resonance. Our forefathers repulsed supernatural threats with such strange-sounding cries: "Avaunt, hell take thee!"; *"Vade retrome, Satana!";* "Dii te averrucent!"; and that most strange of charms, used by Shakespeare (*King Lear* III, iv; *Macbeth* I, iii), and whose origin remains uncertain: "Aroint thee!" The death of infants in their cribs no longer prompts an "Aroint thee!" from the survivors; our age, laconic and partial to abbreviations, prefers "SIDS." Yet its exorcistic significance is clear, for it is hard to suppress the irrational feeling that this form of sudden death is also ascribable to the throttling demon, who is never surprised in its evildoing. Demonologists of past ages inventoried the forms adopted by the Evil One: snake, toad, monk, knight dressed in black, dark cloud and seductive woman. Medical hypotheses in my lifetime suggest different, though equally numerous, natures: parathyroid abnormalities, viral infections, vascular reflexes, nasal occlusion, and more recently, sleep apnea. The nature of SIDS, however, is still undetermined. But it is not pathophysiology that I wish to discuss. My urge now is for venting that stubborn melancholy, that irresoluble puzzlement that explains nothing, but which craves an outlet. For those who have looked at infants' early deaths never cease to ask why, even if they do not expect an answer.

Whoever had it as his lot to be born can account it a sure thing that he must die. Yet the spans of individual life-journeys vary exceedingly. What, then, are we to think of the death of the newly born? Throughout antiquity the sages judged this to be a happy event. *Optimum non nasci,* the best is not to be born. But, if you are born, the next best thing is to exit from this life as expeditiously as you can manage. This pessimistic outlook was the objective appraisal of an age whose worst fault was excessive candor. The old philosophers addressed us directly, as one who talks to a perplexed friend. Why do you insist in treading life's path? Wherever you turn your gaze it is sure to encounter ills and discomfiture: the courts resounding with malisons shouted by litigious parties; the fields forcing on all a harsh, unending toil; the seas and the skies full of dangers. Are you well off? Kiss goodbye forever your peace of mind: uneasiness will keep you company. Poor? Your life will alternate between humiliation and harshness. Married? Count the ills that result from this. But if you remain celibate, you condemn yourself to loneliness. Procreate, and your life will be an unending trial, you will be consumed in the cares that come with nursing and rearing children. Remain without offspring, and survive to woebegoneness. Are you young? You are to be pitied, for your life is unset, and you dwell in ungrateful ignorance and darkness. Old? Pitied twice, for old age is weak *and* forlorn. "What remains to you, if you are not a madman," reads an epigram of uncertain authorship, "is to choose one of these two options: either never to leave the narrow murkiness of the maternal womb, or, once you have been expelled therefrom, go submerge yourself in the gloominess of the Styx." The ancients, like none who followed, perceived the inherent calamitousness of human life. "Of all living beings that breathe the vital air or ramp on the ground, none more miserable than man." And Plautus, with sober finality: "To have lived is preferable to living."

The pessimism of the learned probably did not reach the masses. The common people held life preferable to nonexistence with that unabashed enthusiasm that merited, more than once, the Stoics' contempt. Some peoples, however, may have been sensitive to the philosophers' theorizing. If we are to be-

lieve Herodotus, whose credibility is always in question, a Thra-
cian tribe, the Trausi, developed a ceremonial in perfect consonance with the pessimistic outlook. Upon the birth of an infant,
the family members gathered around the cradle and mourned
the unhappy event. A recitation of the whole catalog of human
sorrows was included in this peculiar custom. In contrast, when
somebody died, the prescribed observance called for banquets
and festivities; and amidst the merriment and rejoicing, there
came a recitation of the ills that the departed had escaped.

The early Christians' view took a completely different turn.
Life is a precious gift from God. What to think, then, of infants' early deaths? Gregory of Nyssa thought of the following
simile. Suppose a banquet of extraordinary richness and abun-
dance is being prepared. Let the man who presides over the
banquet be someone gifted with the knowledge of what
viands are most suited to the temperament and constitution of
each guest. The president of the board ensures that those inclined to tippling be promptly taken away from the banquet,
before becoming drunk; that those who would overindulge in
dainties noxious to their health be removed from the feast;
that those who would take the wrong food be prevented from
lingering over the table furnished with the instruments of
their destruction. Now, those expelled from the banquet
would naturally feel inclined to charge the president with injustice. But if they were to catch a sight of those already beginning to misbehave themselves "in the way of vomitings,
and putting their heads on the table, and unseemly talk," perhaps they would reconsider and be grateful that they had
been spared the effects of this debauch. Thus, the illustration
is clear. Life's board is crowded with savory, sweet, salty, bitter, and pungent foods; not all on it is honey. The Arranger of
the Feast of Life is God's Providence, which withdraws from
the banquet those who, had they been allowed to stay, would
have plunged into debauch. This premise is important. Gregory insists that we accept it. For nothing happens without
God, and, by the same token, "God's dispensations have no

element of chance and confusion in them." A blind, unmeaning occurrence cannot be the work of God.

It would have been better for Gregory to leave us with the helpless exclamation of the Apostle: "O the depth of the riches both of the wisdom and the knowledge of God! How unsearchable are His judgments, and His ways past finding out! For who hath known the mind of the Lord?" (Rom. 11:33–34). Instead, he finds excuses for making inquiries, and nerves himself to sally forth in search of answers. And the result of his meditations is Providence-as-prophylaxis: it is a sign of the divine perfection that not only can existing maladies be cured, but that some are prevented from ever developing. Out of love for us, He who knows the future equally with the past manages to forestall evils that otherwise would inevitably come to pass. And one should not question how it is, then, that those who live wickedly survive. Gregory's subtle counterargument is two-pronged. Either God, in kindness to those who have served him over generations, removes a new member of that family that *would have* stained the immaculate record, or, if no such antecedent exists, nothing authorizes us to doubt His foreknowledge, and to accept that by causing early deaths He removes beings that "would have plunged into a vicious life with a more desperate vehemence than any of those who have actually become notorious for their wickedness."[10]

The Divine Providence as M.C. at the feast of life! And who is to say that Gregory was wrong? But the present era is no longer interested in direct proof or refutation of such arguments. It is no longer the meaning, but the mechanism of early deaths that matters. We should persuade ourselves that it is a sign of maturity that questions about the "whys" are asked less and less, except by young children before school age. Intelligent adults ask how, when, where, and, in particular, how much. Nevertheless, SIDS continues to be an elusive demon. All the enquiries have failed to clarify the nature of the demon's evildoing. Research into the circumstances surrounding these fatalities continues unabated, and through it the modern physician resembles those of his predecessors that dreamed of correlating the visible manifestations of the universe with illness and death. It is reported that in ancient China, during the Chou dynasty, medical men attempted the incredible feat of correlating individual disease with as many natural phenomena as the mind could conceive in the capacity of promoters of illness. If a patient had a fever on a certain day, it could be inferred, by a subtle train of thought, that it was relevant for understanding the disease to know the day of the patient's birth, the season of his marriage, whether the moon was full when sickness struck, and so on. But the number of possible correlations became infinite, and as new ones appeared it became clear that many stood in blatant contradiction with previously established ones. Medicine's reputation was at stake, since medical men were apt to make contradictory pronouncements. To save face, Chinese physicians began to enunciate medical axioms in progressively more abstract terms, until, at last, medicine became indistinguishable from philosophy: it lost its character as a branch of knowledge with practical utility. And this, notes with irony the pathologist-historian G. Majno, was disastrous, for "to a patient with diarrhea there are more pressing concerns than to be instructed in the proper way to conduct his life according to the Tao."

This, we can rest assured, will not happen again. Contemporary medicine will never again lose sight of its pragmatic ends. Yet it is not a small irony that the demon of SIDS has forced modern researchers into resuming the ways of the ancient Chou physicians. Reading the work of epidemiologists one gathers that it has been considered important to discern whether infants who succumb to the "syndrome" of sudden and unexplained death die during the day or at night (most die between midnight and nine A.M.); whether the victim lay prone or supine (most rested on their abdomen); whether the child was legitimate or illegitimate (most are out-of-wedlock); whether death occurred in the cold or in the warm season (most die in winter); whether on a weekend or during weekdays (data are inconsistent). Race, sex, maternal age, birth order, meteorological conditions, time of day—all are thought to be "significant" correlations. Just so, in a remote past, Asian medicine believed it important for prognostication to know whether the patient faced East or West; whether the ailment struck on a clear day or under overcast skies, and whether, when the physician approached the patient, the road was crossed by oxen, or the skies were coursed by a flock of ravens.

Our Predaceous Nature

Some twenty or thirty years ago, an Italian film documentary shocked audiences by the simple expedient of showing the fare that is consumed throughout the world. With a gift for the sensational that must be an inborn trait in *paparazzi,* the filmmakers toured the back kitchens of this earth. In the Far East, the cameras recorded scenes of snakes being skinned while still endowed with undulating motion, then tied into neat vertical bunches, like belts in our department stores, and, at last, consumed eagerly by approving customers. The next scene was filmed inside an expensive Manhattan restaurant, which might have passed for the banquet hall of Sardanapalus. Here, tuxedoed waiters served their moneyed patrons heaps of daintily prepared ants—chocolate covered, the voice behind the screen informed us, and at several hundred dollars a serving for two. The slow-motion footage of spoons dipping into crumbling monticules of small, six-legged creatures of segmented body, then ladling these into the open mouths of delighted revelers, never failed to elicit a murmur of astonishment in the crowd of movie-watchers. Young, and all but blasé about what seemed plain aberrance of the eating function, I joined in the general astonishment. I should not have. For I was familiar with the rural Mexican custom of eating the now famous *"maguey* worm" (actually the larva of a butterfly, *Aegiale hesperialis,* that lives in the leaves of the *maguey,* or agave plant), and had even tried, not without trepidation, a morsel or two. But all this, it must be owned, happened in more innocent times. Since then, suburban hostesses have tendered me the *gusano de maguey,* canned for export, at two North American cocktail parties, at least, one of them as far north as Canada. I do not claim expertise, but it seems to me that the product suffers in the canning and exporting process. Paraphrasing the wine connoisseurs, I might say that "it does not travel well." But then, one must allow, how else would a worm get to travel?

Nor can insect-eating be dealt with in an entirely jocular vein. None other than a cousin of Christ, St. John the Baptist, sustained himself on a strict diet of insects and insect products. At least for the time he preached in Judea, "his food was locusts and wild honey" (Matt. 3:4). And when the Lord spelled out to Moses and Aaron the rules and regulations of approved and disapproved edibles, his divine decree included locusts, grasshoppers, katydids and crickets in the O.K. list, whereas permission for eating other insects was withheld, pending further testing, we assume. Reads the ban in vivid, if zoologically inaccurate style: ". . . all other winged insects that have four legs are loathsome to you" (Lev. 11:20–23). An insect product, honey, was sung by the poets of antiquity; Grecian scholars tell us that it was a component of the ambrosia that delighted the pagan gods at Olympus. But it is not only from the tales of pagans that we acknowledge insect products as ingredients of heavenly-ordained cookery. A professor of zoology at Hebrew University in Jerusalem maintained that the Biblical manna that rained on the Israelites was also an insect product.[1] It was, in his view, the sweetish secretion elaborated by plant lice, or aphids, that suck the sap of plants; because of the rapid evaporation that takes place in the desert, the honeydew secretion is solidified, becoming hard and granular. *Man,* an Arabic term, designates both the aphids and their product; the latter is sold in huge quantities as *man-es-simma,* or manna from the sky, in markets throughout the Arab world, for the preparation of desserts. The tamarisk manna is abundant in the area of Sinai where scholars believe the Exodus took place, and is particularly abundant in that part of the year during which the Exodus is thought to have occurred. Moreover, the Biblical manna fell at night and was collected in the morning (Exod. 16:14–21); and it is especially at night that, free from the hostility of competing ants, the aphids most actively elaborate their sweet juice, the honeydew product that is common to many plant lice.

This illustrious lineage will do little to overcome our current prejudice. The prophets' injunctions, difficult as they are to follow, we profess to obey; the admonitions of the apostles, however stern, we take into our hearts with contrite air. But to imitate St. John the Baptist's dietary habits? This we will not do. Only by rare exception have human societies taken to the class Insecta with as much relish as Westerners today take to beef. Marston Bates, biologist and raconteur, described the selling of bags of toasted leaf-cutting ants in a tropical South American town where he lived for some time.[2] This collation was sold, when in season, at the movie theater, "where it took the place, both in quality and function, of the American popcorn." In another area of the world, he tells us, a tourist wandering into a café was startled by the crunching sound that each of his steps produced as he walked on innumerable locusts' legs with which the floor was strewn. Customers consuming this delicacy were in the habit of discarding the legs and casually throwing them on the floor.

Experts contend that hunger in the world would be much alleviated if human societies could be made to erase their alimentary prejudices.[3] But, go and try to contravene them, if you wish to experience the pain and frustration that prejudice can inflict! Take, for instance, the anti-pig prejudice. In the Middle East, as is well known, Moslems and Jews alike have long detested pork. But the millenarian detestation has been deeper and more widespread than is commonly assumed. In Egypt, swine were thought so unclean at the time of Herodotus (484?–

424? B.C.), that their mere touch was repugnant, let alone their consumption as food. If a man happened to brush himself against one by pure accident, he would run to the Nile and plunge in without undressing, so urgent did he perceive the need to cleanse himself of impurities. When Jews were being systematically Hellenized, the conqueror Antiochus Epiphanes (*c.* 215–163 B.C.) pressured the people to sacrifice swine and eat pork. The scribe Eleazar, forced to place the abhorred meat in his mouth, spat it out with revulsion and declared with the stirring accent of martyrs that he would sooner die than swallow. Consider now, by way of contrast, the cooking of China, where pork has been enjoyed since the Neolithic period with an undisguised partiality that abides in our day. The relatively small Moslem minority there strove to keep up porcine detestation, but without success even though they avoided the very word "pig," using such euphemistic derogation as "the black one." The massive numbers of the Chinese majority prevailed. Their eager enthusiasm transformed this land into the country with the most pigs: 114,000,000 by the last count of which I have knowledge. The massive Indian subcontinent, which has the only comparable demographic concentration, had only four million at that time. It is fair to assume that the *discovery of roast pig* must have taken place in a way similar to that described by Charles Lamb in his humorous essay; for pork continues to exert its fascination, even though sweet-and-sour sauces hide from the contemporary Chinese palate whatever sapid rawness first caught the fancy of the Neolithic ancestors. The Chinese character for "home" is composed of the ideogram that represents "roof," with the one that represents "pig" placed underneath; this should suffice to convince anyone that the pig has earned a prominent place in the nation's heart—before, that is, being assigned to its final place of residence, the stomach. Nevertheless, it remains puzzling that a society that prides itself on having invented a cuisine that renders palatable all that nature made digestible (and much that, on first thought, might appear not to be), continues to turn a squeamish mien toward dairy products. When a sizable portion of the world's population derives both delight and protein from milk and milk products, many Chinese continue to deem it ludicrous that a grown person should persist in such indulgence after being weaned. The mere sight of an American milkshake can elicit in some Chinese the violent revulsion that Americans reserve for a dish of reptiles, or grasshoppers, these perfectly legitimate foods whose nutritive value is fully utilized in many parts of the world.

I like to imagine that, aside from the blocks imposed by the mind, nothing in the universe would be rejected by man's undiscriminating stomach. Vegetal, animal, or mineral. Given reasonable evolutionary time, we would evolve the enzymes needed to disintegrate stainless steel, or to digest cast iron, if such dietary whims ever appeared and became inveterate. In Java, pregnant women are known to consume blocks of white clay; and not long ago, a similar earthy clay, shaped into figurines, palliated the hunger of the dispossessed in Peru and Bolivia. And not only does extreme want compel the hungry to seek unorthodox nourishment. Excess, too, leads the appetite astray, or as Disraeli put it, "gluttony produces monsters, and turns away from nature to feed on unwholesome meats." For virtually *all* is game to omnivorous man, whose predaceous nature is expressed through the mouth. Of all parts of the body, this is the one that most graphically betokens our tendency to imperialism and domination; it is through the mouth that the external world is grasped, seized, and turned into the same stuff as ourselves. And since this avocation goes back to protohistory, it is not surprising that the mouth should have evolved the finest set of cutlery—teeth—with which to pierce, tear, and grind a stubbornly unmalleable nonself. Stimulate the cheeks of a sweet, innocent newborn infant, just out of the maternal womb: he will respond with the "sucking-clinging reflex," the brief enactment of that obscure atavic drive by which our predaceous nature would have us clasp, fasten down, and devour a prey.

Perhaps nothing reveals more strikingly the overwhelming orality of our species, than to confirm, by firsthand observation, the heterogeneity of objects recovered from the alimentary tract, during life or posthumously. Coins, pens, watches, fragments of shoes and other garments, nails, pens, toothpicks, astonishing lengths of metallic wire and assorted jewelry; these things form only a partial list. And it were naive to dismiss the prodigious nature of the finding on the grounds that such ingestions are often accidental, or the erratic act of a deranged mind. For this would be tantamount to denying the two most valuable tenets of unbiased experience: that there is no such thing as a wholly random human act, and that there is much to learn from deviancy, by those willing to listen.

And then, sometimes, it is the prodigious that comes the observer's way. One afternoon, when as a pathologist-in-training I made the inventory of the surgical specimens received in the laboratory that day—from the innocuous birthmark removed as a concession to the patient's vanity, to the acutely diseased viscus urgently removed under life-threatening circumstances—my task was interrupted by the arrival of a young surgeon bringing with him one more specimen. "A tumor of the stomach," he said, as he unfolded the surgical towels and looked at me with a sly smile on his face. What he uncovered was a large mass of long black hairs densely matted together, covered by a viscid, glaring substance. Not a pleasant sight; and a foul odor, probably due to incompletely digested food particles trapped within the hairy mass, rendered it still more intimidating. Yet I cannot describe the strange object in less offensive ways: it was a large mass of entangled black hairs, weighing nearly two pounds, compressed into a shape reminiscent of a stomach, whence it had been extracted, and covered by a slimy, fetid fluid. The all too visible craftiness of my surgeon friend at last gave way to a sensible desire to instruct the confused neophyte. We were in front of a *bezoar,* I was informed. More precisely, a bezoar made of hair, or *trichobezoar,* found in the stomach of a pale adolescent girl. She had complained of vague abdominal pains for a few months; a tender, mobile mass could be palpated in her abdomen. The mass now lay before us, and, as I was to learn subsequently, deserved more than the hurried glance of queasiness commingled with anxiety that I condescended to grant it. For despite its repulsive appearance, this object was the individual member of a class that has been much revered, and was once treasured by the powerful.[4]

In effect, scholars trace the term "bezoar" to the Arabic *badzehr* or Persian *padzahr,* meaning "counterpoison," for it was once believed that certain solid objects found inside the stomach of mammals possessed curative properties. The Oriental bezoar, recovered from the fourth stomach of goats *(Capra aegagrus),* or gazelles, in Syria and Persia, was much valued; its magical aura was no little enhanced by its Oriental provenance. In time, the West, too, furnished a source of these mysterious remedial stones. The stomach of the vicuña sheep *(Auchenia vicunna)* is known to harbor them. And although modern researchers are of the opinion that these concretions represent precipitates of bile components and cholesterol salts, men of past ages held different, most singular beliefs. To Emperor Charles V of Spain, they were magic stones that rid him of the morbid thoughts that tormented him. Edward IV of England survived the effects of a poisoned wound thanks to the beneficent emanations of one bezoar of his property. And after the advent of James I to the English throne, the official in charge of making an inventory of the crown jewels described "also one great Bezoar stone, set in goulde, that was Queen Elizabeth's, with some Unicorne's horn, in a paper; and some other large Bezoar stone, broken in pieces, delivered to our own hands by Lord Brooke." The less fortunate, unable to own their private bezoar encased in gold and adorned with emeralds, did not fall beyond the pale of what today's bureaucrats identify with the execrable term of "health-delivery system": apothecaries concerned with the public weal loaned bezoars to the public, on lease, for a weekly or monthly fee.

As to the human bezoar of my experience, its origin was

altogether different, though no less remarkable. It had formed by gradual accretion of undigestible hairs, swallowed habitually. Nervous girls (trichobezoars are especially prevalent in young girls) may fall prey to this compulsion, just as other persons bite their nails, or engage in diverse kinds of automatic, regressive behavior. Thus, we find a sort of mania, a nervous manipulation of the body, at the origin of the bezoar. A pretty girl coquettishly twirls the tips of her braids around her finger, haply bringing them close to her lips; or, perhaps, the beauty holds a lock of hair between her pearly teeth, a gesture that seems to enhance the piquancy of her smile. But now and then she bites, and swallows. And she may experience a titillating sensation as the hair fragment travels down to her stomach. Yes; let no one be surprised to learn that it was the pleasurable sensation of a slow deglutition that she found most habit-forming. Recall that one of the convives in the Satyricon confessed that he often wished he had a crane's neck, so as to prolong the duration of this feeling. But, in the end, hair is added unto hair, the mass slowly grows, lingers inexplicably within the stomach, whose sluggish motions gradually compact the growing mass . . . and the trichobezoar is complete. From the day I saw the astonishing specimen I have not been able to look at feminine hair without feeling strangely troubled. Botticelli's Venus, with her long mane of hair agitating in the wind, or Gustave Moreau's mysterious women, whose hair drags on the ground, are disquieting. But it is the luscious treatment of female hair by some of the so-called Symbolist painters (for instance, in the *Eve* of Lucien Lévy-Dhurmer, where flaming red locks of hair are seen crowding the mouth of a somewhat anemic, British-looking first woman) that inevitably raises the question: "Did she eat it?" And I suspect that even children's stories are seen in a new light by those who come under the spell of the bezoar. Surgeons describing a long trichobezoar, which extended from the stomach several feet into the intestine, came up with a new technical term: "Rapunzel syndrome."

To the massive variety of ingesta must correspond an equally varied panoply of "gastric images"—that is, of mental representations of the stomach. Psychiatrists have yet to explore the massive array. The Hindu and the Buddhist, who link vegetarianism to a respect for animal life, must fear the stomach as a potential repository of base passions: the stomach as the seat of evil. Mahatma Gandhi, however, attempted to eat meat, believing, he wrote, "that it was good, that it would make me strong and daring and that, if the whole country took to meat-eating, the English could be overcome." The stomach as the seat of combativeness: an idea that was once seriously upheld. It was Bernard Shaw, I think, who derided it with customary wit: the bull is a strict vegetarian, yet it counts itself among the fiercest of all animals. Gandhi's attempt, in any case, was a total failure; he choked on every bite, was tormented by nightmares, and felt "as though a live goat were bleating inside [him]." Most of all, he was pained at the thought of the shame that he would experience if his father and mother were to see him as a transgressor, a meat-eater. The stomach as the portal of shame. Those who shun "unclean" animals are perhaps haunted by visions of carcasses decomposing by the roadside, putrefying in the sun; perhaps they shudder to think that the interior of the body might be made to house such filth. The stomach as cesspool. What dimly conscious idea may have surged in the mind of the patient whom I once saw swallowing nails, screws, and wire? Perhaps her disturbed psyche conceived the stomach as an organ with the power to triturate, to mill, to pulverize. For such an idea is not alien to sane minds; it has, in fact, precedent among the learned, though it were folly to equate the learned with the sane. In the early era of the study of gastric physiology, a Scottish physician, Archibald Pitcairn, calculated the crushing power of the stomach. He did not do this by direct experimentation, Heaven forbid, but by a fine inference, which showed amply the robust nature of his sanity. He took Borelli's estimate of the force that can be exerted by the flexor muscles of the thumb, and after weighing these muscles he weighed the muscles of the stomach and abdominal wall. Comparing these weights he reached the astonishing conclusion that the stomach can exert a compressive force of 400,000 pounds! The stomach as grinder. The learned have put forth theories that surpass in absurdity the wildest speculations of the ignorant. Chemists and physiologists have maintained that the degradation of foodstuffs in the stomach is chiefly owed to fermentation, to heat, to concoction, to material effervescence, and the like.[5]

In these days of food faddism, dieting, waist consciousness, body building, youth worship, and assorted modes of metaphysics through ingestion and philosophies of consumption, the words of the illustrious Scottish scientist William Hunter seem to acquire a new meaning. Said Hunter, addressing a group of disgruntled physiologists who argued over their pet hypotheses to explain the gastric function: "Some physiologists will have it, that the stomach is a mill, others, that it is a fermenting vat, others, again, that it is a stew-pan; but, in my view of the matter, it is neither a mill, a fermenting vat, nor a stew-pan; but a stomach, gentlemen, a stomach."[6,7]

THE SOMETIMES PERMITTED

All is potential food to our predaceous nature. And yet, the canonical code of civilization consigns one clear prohibition: man must not feed on man. The taboo is ancient and unambiguous. So long as society has seemed worthy of calling itself civilized, it has held that only barbarism and fury can explain the aberrant instances of men finding human flesh appetible, as do wolves, bears, and tigers. Extreme hunger, however, is an exception. Chrysippus and Zeno, who taught impassiveness in the face of misfortune, sanctioned nonetheless the use of human carcasses as food, when by this means death by famine could be avoided.

There are some examples, perhaps too well known, of this extremity. A band of hardy explorers survived at Donner Pass after eating two Indians that one of the group, mad with hunger, had murdered. The survivors were comforted by society's compassion, and admitted to the annals of heroism of American Western expansion. A party of French settlers on their way to the colony of Senegal, irresponsibly left on a raft at sea during a shipwreck, survived (fifteen survivors, more than a hundred dead) for about two weeks under the scalding African sun, by putting the sick to death and eating them. They were immortalized by Géricault in his magnificent and large canvas *The Raft of the Medusa,* which one admires today at the Louvre. A team of Uruguayan rugby players, stranded in the Andean peaks when the airplane in which they traveled crashed on October 12, 1972, survived for weeks by resorting to cannibalism. They tried to cook the flesh of the dead, but there was little fuel, and they had to eat it mostly raw. It is reported that, when the rescuers arrived and tried to identify the dead, one survivor tossed a skull to another and said, in an elated accent that horrified the rescuers: "You should know who this guy is; you ate his brains!" But society was again generous in receiving those who had just come from such a harrowing ordeal. The young survivors were mainly pupils or former pupils of a Catholic school run by Irish churchmen; thus their insistence in finding a theologic justification for their distressing answer to the problem of survival. In a pronouncement that gave new tension to individual faiths slackened by this gruesomeness, a theologian at Rome said that their action had been "only apparently cannibalistic," and that the need to survive superseded all negative elements of their behavior. Nevertheless the young survivors asseverated, in front of a crowd of journalists in Montevideo, that the harsh test they had endured did not set them in conflict with their Christian beliefs. "Christ offered his flesh and blood for men to consume," said one of them in a somewhat strained theological parallel, "giving us to understand that we must do the same." Others found this expression felicitous, and hurried to contribute embellishments, whereby cannibalism was made to accord with the doctrinal corpus of the Church.[8]

Mere multiplication of the examples would not help us to

throw a new light on this behavior. But it is a fact that vast numbers of people, if placed under like conditions, will behave in the same way. Whole armies, like Napoleon's in its disastrous Russian campaign, will choose to use fallen comrades as a source of protein when nothing else avails. Whole towns, in the maddening privation imposed by drought, spoliation, and war, will turn to the identical relief. In the siege of Paris during the religious wars of the sixteenth century, the hungry population first exhausted the hoarded grain; then sacrificed horses, asses, cats and dogs; then hunted for rats in the sewers; then ate the tallow in candles, the soap, the leather of gloves, purses and shoes. In the extremity of despair, many ate the flesh of those who had succumbed to famine, and shortly before the siege was lifted bands of the famished were seen disinterring corpses from their graves, in a desperate attempt to find something to eat. The chronicler L'Estoile says that of the ground bones of skeletons a dough was prepared with which a bread was made. Noting that starvation did not blight the sense of humor of Parisians, he tells us that this preparation was dubbed "the bread of *la Montpensier*," in quaint allusion to an unpopular lady of those times. "All who ate it, died," adds the chronicler with the intent of exemplariness. Closer to us—too close to be smoothed by the ironies of a contemporary L'Estoile—are the chilling narratives of similar horrors of recent memory. In World War II, the siege of Stalingrad alone could supply to the modern chronicler a quota of horror in no way inferior to the worst ever unleashed by the savagery of man.

THE FORBIDDEN

There are only two themes worth writing or reading about: love and death, *eros* and *thanatos*. And if the pressures of our time, sloth, or inertia, should force us to be compendious, we could do with one theme only, cannibalism—decoction, synthesis, repository and subsumption of the other two.

Cannibalism is *thanatos* in pure form, the elemental and most ancient form of aggression. What greater injury to a foe than to devour him? His hands will be choice bits, reserved to the leaders, as was the custom among Polynesian tribes; his entrails torn out, as was done by sacrificers of the Leopard Society in Sierra Leone, who inserted their hands through gashes in the victim's abdomen and pulled out his liver and intestines; his blood drunk in his presence, as did the Scythians according to Herodotus; or tongues pulled out with fishhooks, severed, roasted, and eaten in front of the unfortunates, as reported of Fijian cannibals, with taunts of "We are eating your tongues!" shouted to the victims. But cannibalism is also *eros*, unbelievable as it may seem for so cruel and ferocious a practice. Scholars have remarked a fundamental ambivalence in cannibalistic aggression: not all members of the tribe took part in eating the flesh of the slain, and elaborate rituals were set up: ritual protection of the killer; ceremonies connected with the consumption of the flesh; rules applying to what may be eaten and by whom; and even the taking of the name of the eaten by the eater, or the bestowing of the name of the victim on the slayer's offspring. In the Freudian interpretation, ritual is a way to deal with ambivalence. And the ambivalence of cannibalism was so striking that students of societies in which this loathsome practice prevailed were led to conclude that strands of affection appeared curiously interwoven with the most heartless expressions of individual and collective sadism.[9]

Eli Sagan, author of a psychoanalytic study of cannibalism, spoke of "affectionate cannibalism," in which feelings of affection are manifested toward the object of aggression, in such a way that the boundaries of *eros* and *thanatos,* so neat upon superficial canvassing of their respective jurisdictions, lose their sharpness.[10] The eating of kinsmen, which early explorers did not disassociate from other forms of cannibalism, is clearly the primitive expression of a desire to perpetuate a relationship with the departed. A sublimated version of this desire is expressed by the civilized person who carries in a brooch a lock of hair of the departed, or who places a small quantity of ashes in an urn. The primitive man makes a collar with the bones, or a baldric with the skin, and wears them on his person. Incapable of metaphors, he enacts the movements of his psyche with chilling concreteness. Of a cannibal who had eaten a kinsman, it was reported that he made arrows with the bones, which he carried with him; and everywhere he went he used to say, "my brother and I," without even looking at his quiver. Such is the tenor of inner life in all members of the human species. During infancy, separation from the sources of love and sustenance is not followed by quiet dejection; a reaction to this frustration is always active and always aggressive. We react with anger, and it is not difficult to accept the analysts' interpretation that we conceive the idea, however ill-formed or unconscious, of eating the person who has abandoned us. The cannibal goes beyond the acceptance of a metaphoric satisfaction of his anger by an act of "oral incorporation"; he lives it literally.

Before the Freudian era, the complexity of the cannibal's mind went unappreciated; cannibalism was no more than a perversion of the appetite joined to a specifically human mode of fury. Montaigne was among the first to make distinctions and to set forth, as it were, two moral categories of anthropophagy. He listens, astonished, to the tales of sailors returning from *"la France antarctique"* (Brazil) and concludes that "there is nothing barbarous in that nation, from what I hear, but each one calls barbarism what is not his own usage. . . . In them, the natural virtues and properties are alive and vigorous that we have bastardized here, out of our wish to accommodate them to the pleasure of our corrupt tastes" (Book 1, chap. 31). Here we have Rousseau's noble savage, all in one piece, prefigured before his official arrival. Then, coming to grips with ritual cannibalism, Montaigne is careful to note that if those peoples practice the eating of human flesh, "it is not, as some may think, to nourish themselves, as the Scythians used to do; *it is in order to represent an extreme vengeance.*" The new taxonomy had only awaited this precise formulation: there is brutish, quasi-animal anthropophagy, which is purely gastronomical, and there is that practiced "for the purpose of representing an extreme form of vengeance."

Preoccupation with a moral dimension of cannibalism is, in fact, much older than Montaigne. A rich literature exists in which the victim is not regarded merely as undifferentiated food. In the earliest myths, the victim often is not even the direct target of an "extreme vengeance," but a vehicle through which the latter is foisted on a third party. Atreus's revenge calls for the votive massacre of the sons of Thyestes; then, the tender limbs of the immolated children are minced, boiled in a bronze cauldron, carefully dressed, and served to the unsuspecting father in a deceptive feast of reconciliation. The blood, mixed with wine, eddies away from Thyestes' lips when he brings the cup toward his mouth. The sun arrests its course in the sky, as if horrified by the imminence of the impious repast. But all these prodigies are useless: Thyestes swills and guzzles, the fierce Atreus reveals to him what he has eaten, and this most frightful of tragedies ends amidst the cries of horror of the wretched father, mad with pain. And from Atreus's quaking table issues forth a long line of "extreme revenges" in the gastronomical mode. Having offended a Persian king, the unwitting Harpagus is served a dish prepared from the flesh of his own sons, and is asked repeatedly whether the meat is to his liking. At the end of the macabre banquet, the king orders the heads brought in and presented to the unsuspecting father. Asked, then, what he thought of the meal, Harpagus uttered a reply that the Stoics adduced as proof that reason can have complete dominion over passion. "At the king's table no dish can displease," is all he managed to say. And more was not needed. He could have howled in pain as an outraged father, says a Stoic philosopher, but as a father there was nothing he could do. What did he achieve by maintaining his calm in the face of this hideous sadism? To be excused from dessert, I suppose: he had other sons to think of.

This form of gastronomical revenge persists for centuries. On the fourth day of his storytelling, Boccaccio recounts the true story of Sieur Guillaume de Roussillon, who killed his wife's lover, took out his heart, had the cook "make thereof an excellent ragout," and fed it to his wife. Sorrow-stricken, but seemingly unrepentant, the good lady threw herself from a high window to her death below. In another story of the Decameron (fifth day, 8), that of Nastagio degli Onesti, revenge takes an unexpected turn: the heart of the unpitying woman is fed to the dogs, thus consummating what a scholar termed "anthropophagy by proxy." In Shakespeare's *Titus Andronicus*, a logic of sorts can be perceived in the cannibalistic vengeance. The evildoers are baked into a pie, "whereof their mother daintily hath fed/Eating the flesh that she herself hath bred" (V, iii, 61–62). The murderous impulse attempts to reestablish a former order: it returns to the abdomen what had issued therefrom. This is the logic of passion, if I may be excused the absurd expression. The fact is, the same aggression has been used toward the father. A tabloid published at Troyes in 1608 displayed a front page that yielded nothing to the shrillest headlines of our *National Enquirer.* It read: "Prodigious history of a young maiden of Dole, in Franche-Comté, who fed the liver of her newborn son to the young Gentleman that had abused her modesty under cover of a dissembled marriage; including how she made him die with cruelty, and placed herself in the hands of Justice to receive an exemplary punishment: Saturday, the 19th day of November, 1608. With the sentence of the Parliamentary Court pronounced against her."[11]

The theme of vengeful cannibalism knows no boundaries. The Chinese, who chose to elevate filial piety to the status of a cardinal virtue for longer than anyone cares to guess, spawned nonetheless their peculiar versions of the banquet of Atreus. An ancient chronicle, known as the *History of East Chou's Many States,* gives interesting examples. One took place during the conquest of the principality of Jung Shan (406 B.C.) and is described below.[12]

Yue Yang, a valorous general, is in charge of the military

operations. He has set siege to the capital, and is about to start an offensive, when he is informed that his son is inside the city. The besieged prince profits from this circumstance to try to dissuade his fearful enemy. A parley is arranged at which the general's son, at the head of a retinue, meets his father outside the city walls. The general is unmoved. Arbalest at the shoulder, and in full combat regalia, he thunders against the young man, upbraiding him for having chosen to cast his lot with an unprincipled ruler, and for being one of those who "know not when to stay and when to leave." ["Now he tells him!" writes a commentator in a sanguine marginal note.]

"Take these words to your master," Yue Yang says to his son, "with my summons for his immediate surrender."

"What the prince will decide to do next I cannot guess," stutters the young man, unable to file either horn of his dilemma. "But I beg you, as your son, to hold your attack for a while, that I may have some time to try to persuade him to accept your orders."

"It will not be said that Yue Yang is impervious to the words of a son who appeals to him in the name of the bond of love that links father and son. For this alone I postpone my attack for one month, and one month only."

The fierce ardor and impatience of Yue Yang were proverbial. That his hand had been stayed by his son's plea was an extraordinary achievement, and one that infused new hope in the besieged. So long as Yue Yang's son was hostage, they thought, all was not lost. At the end of the truce a new parley is arranged, in which offers of money, honors, and dignities are made to the general. All without effect. But a new postponement of the assault is obtained. And at the end of this term, a new reprieve again is granted.

Three months elapse, while the besiegers, arrayed for battle, must be content with intercepting marauders and keeping a watch over the city gates. Three months, during which the courtly intrigue at Yue Yang's headquarters intensifies ominously. Disquieting rumors reach the Duke of Wei, who had sent Yue Yang specific orders to take the city with the greatest possible despatch. Why does Yue Yang remain inactive, ask the courtiers. His troops are far superior to the enemy's. The delay demoralizes the attackers, and increases the chances that succor come to the besieged, after all. And to these speeches, uttered in ways carefully calculated to reach the Duke of Wei's ears, are added letters that viciously accuse the general of placing his paternal feelings above his obligations to his country. The Duke of Wei makes no reply. He places the letters in a secret cabinet and writes to the general: "I support your strategy."

When, at last, Yue Yang and his forces close in on the city, the defenders are well prepared. Months of postponement of the attack have allowed the fortification of defenses, the raising of parapets, the buttressing of walls, and the introduction of victuals. For a while the issue seems dubious, but soon the attackers' might is felt in all its terror. The defenders' chief military commander is killed with an arrow shot that pierces his skull, and this misfortune obligates the prince of Jung Shan to implement an emergency plan. Yue Yang's son is tied with ropes to a long pole, hoisted over the battlements, and placed in full sight of the attackers. With pitiful cries he asks to be spared, and implores both sides to show mercy. The troops that clamber on improvised scaffolding fall back upon recognizing, in the bundled-up victim, their own general's son. But Yue Yang is inflexible, and makes ready to shoot the first arrow at his son. This dreadful act is prevented by the promptness with which the besieged haul the unfortunate young man to safety, while others cover the operation with volleys of darts, stones, and arrows flung from machicolations. The young man is untied, and despondently drags himself to his prince, at whose feet he avows, rather redundantly, the futility of his efforts to calm his father's wrath. For all answer he is handed a sword, with which he commits suicide.

A conclave now takes place among high military officers. The collapse of Jung Shan is imminent, and the most desperate proposals must receive consideration. This last-resort plan is agreed upon by all: the cadaver of Yue Yang's son is to be beheaded; with the remaining fleshy parts, a steamed preparation of culinary merit is to be fixed. This macabre dish is to be sent to Yue Yang. The rationale of the plan is at one and the same time simplicity itself and surfeit of Oriental subtlety. The spectacle of his own son turned into sweet-and-sour morsels, or some such, would be sure to evoke a strong reaction in the general. In theory, this reaction could be of several types. He could die on the spot, of apoplexy. Or he could suffer a convulsive fit. Less severely, he could be seized by some form of furious, irrational, blind rage; or he could fall into a profound depression. The precise nature of the effect mattered little. The important thing was, that his mind would not fail to be conspicuously discomposed. For a man who had thrice agreed to postpone an important siege for the sake of his son could only be a man exquisitely sensitive to the demands of paternal love. And such a man, went the reasoning, after seeing his son in the state to which culinary art had reduced him, would be utterly incapable of leading his troops to the completion of his victory.

A group of envoys, carrying with them the fragrant wicker baskets and the delicately decorated receptacles with their sinister collation, appears before Yue Yang. An elaborate Oriental politeness is not precluded by the nature of their mission:

"Our Lord and Prince humbly asks of your benevolence that you accept these gifts." And, uncovering the large pan with the severed head: "Because your son was unable to discharge his duty with honor, his life was taken away. It is with profound respect that we bring to you his flesh. His wife and children survive him. Our prince commands us to tell you that they, too, shall die, unless you desist from your plans to take Jung Shan."

The chronicle does not record surprise, astonishment or terror. Yue Yang remains impassive. At last, he chides the severed head in these terms:

"Impotent to help your master towards victory, inept to make him accept an honorable surrender, all you did was to whimper and to cry, like a baby who, sucking at the nipple and anxious for baubles, at one and the same time wails and be-smears his cheeks with milk."

And these words are followed by an odious deed, unexampled in the annals of infamy of the entire world. Facing the ambassa-dors, Yue Yang grabs a bowl, fills it with the meat that is pre-sented to him, and with steady pulse—a test of which was his deftness at maneuvering the chopsticks—eats up until the bowl is empty. With a cold gleam in his eyes he addresses the ambas-sadors:

"I will long remember the honor of this offering. Pray tell your master so. Tell him, also, that when I enter the city my first thought will be to thank him in person. I, too, carry precious pots and pans; and excellent cooks accompany me. I shall recip-rocate as my dignity and good manners require me to do."

Having heard the result of his embassy, the prince of Jung Shan did not seem much inclined to wait for the promised retribution. He retired to his bedchamber, and hanged himself.

The wrath of Yue Yang at the sack of Jung Shan was long remembered. But he did not stay long. He left a garrison to secure the place and went back to Wei. The Duke, his master, did him honor, receiving him at the gates and sparing no mark of preferment in his behalf. Answering the endearments of his master, who praised his sacrifice, Yue Yang stated that he be-lieved it had been his duty to prevail over all personal feelings, including "those that a father normally has for his son." A ban-quet was given in his honor, at which wine was offered to him in a golden cup, held by the Duke's hand while the general drank. One more reward was announced at the end of the festivity. A large coffer inlaid with pearls and emeralds was brought into the banquet hall, and transported to the general's house to the crowd's merriment and admiration. That night, Yue Yang opened it expecting to find jewels or valuable objects inside. He found a few documents at the bottom of the coffer. These were the letters that the general's detractors had written in his absence, wherein specious accusations were laid down. As he read through them, Yue Yang realized that he had been disturbingly close to being assassinated; he owed his safety to the unflagging trust that the Duke had shown.

The next day, he went in haste to thank the Duke for a favor whose real magnitude he had just appreciated. "My victory at Jung Shan," said the general, "was something I did at the command and through the inspiration of Your Highness, not unlike the tricks that dogs and horses perform at the bidding of their masters, who train them and support them."

"I alone trusted you," replied the Duke, "but you alone vanquished. You deserve all the honors."

When the celebrations were over, however, peculiar dispositions were taken, the occasion of much gossip and speculation at the palace. Yue Yang was elevated to the post of governor of Lin Shou, but relieved of the command of the army. Astute courtiers, always on the trail of intrigue, inferred from this a hidden intent, perhaps a crafty foresight that meant to contain the growth of power in an ambitious and potentially dangerous man. An officer once asked the Duke:

"Yue Yang had proved his courage and his loyalty. Why did you not use him to defend the border, or allow him to stay at the countryside in this province?"

The Duke smiled, and did not answer. But another officer quickly interjected:

"Yue Yang did not love his son. Can such a man be expected to love his sovereign?"

The episode ends here, but the *History of East Chou's Many States* contains one more variation of the anthropophagic theme. It passes for an authentic episode in the life of Confucius and may be told in few words.

Tse Lu, a disciple of the famous philosopher, has been seriously compromised in the intrigue that surrounds a problematic royal succession. He sides with the losing party, is caught trying to free an important prisoner, and is summarily executed. The man in power, the Duke of Wei, deems it opportune to give Confucius a sobering lesson on the impracticality of philosophers meddling into practical affairs. Although there is no evidence that Confucius directly engaged in seditious activities, the tyrant is convinced that the old man promotes in young people the pernicious and unwholesome habit of thinking for themselves. At any rate, the Duke has learned that opportune intimidation is a policy with much to recommend it. Accordingly, he orders the remains of Tse Lu appropriately condimented, roasted, and sent to Confucius for the now familiar "representation of an extreme vengeance" that we have seen so popularly received in the West, although in this case it was a prophylactic one.

The envoys of the Duke of Wei appear before Confucius, and amidst much bowing and kowtowing, and protestations of humility and service, display "the humble gifts brought as a token of the homage that power owes to wisdom." Confucius hears their words and silently inspects the dishes. At this point, the chronicle states that the meat had been thoroughly ground, from which it is valid to infer that Tse Lu may have looked like an Oriental version of a *pâté de foie;* at any rate, any resemblance to the original likeness would have been purely coincidental. Confucius orders the dishes to be covered, and asks: "Is this the flesh of Tse Lu?"

All are astonished at the sagacity of the philosopher. When, at last, one of the envoys dares to ask how he managed to accomplish what seemed a feat of divination, Confucius is said to have volunteered one piece of the type of common sense that earned him fame: "I saw no reason for the Duke to honor me in this fashion," was his laconic answer.

There was no wit, no figure of speech, no veiled allusion or double meaning by which to return the humiliation. None of those things that we come to expect in such narratives in the West. But of all stories on cannibalism prompted by underhanded depravity, this is the only one in which the presumptive victim sees the trap in the nick of time. Confucius did not touch the baleful repast. He grieved for his pupil, and died three years later, being seventy-three years old at his death.

EPILOGUE

So prominent a place for the gruesome subject of cannibalism in a survey of the human body is not unjustified.[13] Debatable as the researches of modern psychiatry inevitably are, they firmly prove that an overwhelming "orality" colors all spheres of human activity. That this orality comes in all hues of the aggressive is also immediately apparent, for images of anthropophagy rise in our mind, if not in our consciousness, from earliest childhood. If it is true that fairy tales express the things that go on in children's minds, what cannibalistic orgies are dreamt of in the nursery! In the psychoanalytic interpretation that Bruno Bettelheim presented so well,[14] Hansel and Gretel eating up the gingerbread house are symbolically nibbling at their own mother. When the child is only an infant who wakes up hungry in the darkness, he experiences the anguish of fear, hunger, and abandonment or desertion. Later, being weaned, the infant projects onto the mother all the anxiety and frustration felt when she ceases to be the nourishing Mother. And still later, when the child reaches the age at which the language of symbols can be understood, the mention of that gingerbread house brings forth a plethora of the feelings of "oral greediness" that welled up in his inner self. Here, at last, is the passive Mother satisfying the long-repressed, obscure cravings. But one does not devour one's mother with impunity. So that in the midst of their gluttony, Hansel and Gretel are made prisoners of a witch who, notice, is also cannibalistic. According to Bettelheim, the witch personifies "the destructive aspects of orality," with all their dangers, and conflicts, and attending sense of guilt. It will be necessary to triumph over one's own anthropophagic tendencies to become a well-balanced adult. And similar interpretations are possible for many, if not most, fairy tales. The oral symbolism in "Little Red Riding Hood" is too obvious. And the explicit sexual symbolism hardly surprises anyone any more; for as time goes by it becomes increasingly clear that *eros* and *thanatos* are, at bottom, the same "consuming passion."

Normal life courses placidly by, partly in spite of, and largely thanks to, the powerful and destructive oral drive that runs in the underlayers of the self. In disease, the manifestations of its disorder are always spectacular. Orality raging amok pushes patients with mental retardation to ingest nails, wire, coins, pieces of glass, metallic files, and other objects that stagger the imagination. Why do patients with an enzyme deficiency, the Lesch-Nyhan syndrome, literally devour themselves? Prey to an alteration of behavior that is but incompletely explained by their disturbed bodily chemistry, these patients uncontrollably bite their hands, or their lips, inflicting serious wounds of self-mutilation.

God of mercy: if we must live in a world where man devours man, sometimes in metaphor and sometimes in bloody-fanged reality, grant us the strength to endure its violent paroxysms. Give us not the tempestuous fury of Thyestes, which dislocated the sun from its fixed orbit—after his mouth had made him an orphan in the world. Not the strength of Harpagus, which turns the heart to stone, nor that of Yue Yang, which triumphed over the cruelty of hyenas by opposing to it an even harsher cruelty. Give us, rather, that kind of strength that confronts malice with serenity and ill will with clear-sighted understanding. The kind of power granted to Confucius. The restrained, percipient might that deflects men's rancor, and counters their invitation to sit at the banquet of Atreus with a collected, civil, but inflexible: "No, thank you."

The Female Breast

With an Olympian disregard for the platitudinous, *Gray's Anatomy* informs us that breasts are present in all, but that they remain rudimentary in infants, children, and men; only in women of reproductive age do these organs attain their "exquisite development." In the adult nullipara, one discovers on the anterior chest wall, from the second to the sixth or seventh ribs, two eminences that protrude from three to five centimeters anteriorly, and extend between ten and twelve centimeters from top to bottom. O, the objectivity of science! *Gray's Anatomy* will not be drawn into the furious maelstrom of debate that lies behind the relationship of measurements and esthetics. These figures are merely stated, given as scientific fact. The weight of an individual breast of these dimensions, we are told, is 150 to 200 grams, but may increase to 500 grams during lactation.

It will seem equally superfluous, even to the least observant, to add that the shape of these organs can vary. The breast may adopt the likeness of a discoidal, hemispherical, or conical eminence. Keener observation may be required to confirm the true fact that the left is generally larger than the right. But shape is, nonetheless, of the essence in a consideration of anatomy; more so, perhaps, in this region than in others. In the twenty-second

volume of *La Grande Encyclopédie,* an admirable scholarly
undertaking of the savants of Paris in the last century,[1] one
reads additional information on this matter. On superficial examination, the form of the breast strikes the observer as being
quite variable, and having no ethnic significance whatsoever. It
is the case, however, that the heirs of the famed *encyclopédistes*
of the Enlightenment spent considerable effort, and no little of
their science, in pondering how frequently or infrequently a
certain breast shape is found in women of different appearance.
They perceived, then, that the hemispheral form is predominant among brunettes, whereas in blondes the breasts are more
commonly pear-shaped or conical.

The more pronounced a certain somatic type, the more the
reiterative occurrence of breast-shape type. Pyriform shapes in
Mongoloid women are not "natural"—that is, not conformable
to the original allotments of nature. What this might mean for
the concept of feminine beauty in different races is best left
unexplored, for as soon as we tread on the difficult grounds of
esthetics we are left with no definable canon to guide us.
Confining themselves to facts, the sages tell us: pyriform outlines in the referred circumstance should be *prima facie* evidence of racial mixture. And they are equally dogmatic in other
areas: Black women, they say, manifest just as much tendency
to adhere to a morphologic stereotype. "Their breasts are conical and pendulous. Thanks to the great laxity of the subcutaneous tissue and the elastic framework, they can be so lengthened
as to allow mothers to nurse babies strapped to their backs."
Indeed, massage, stretching, and the plasticity of tissues bring
about startling results. "Women [of certain primitive tribes] can
pass their breasts underneath the axilla, and have them come
to touch each other on their backs."

A relation of the external anatomy of what standard English
used to call, until the mid-nineteenth century, "woman's
charms," is easily completed. Not at the exact center of this
organ, but somewhat below it, a small cylindrical or conical
body rises from the center of a pigmented and somewhat

roughened circle of skin. It is the *papilla mammae*, or nipple, usually corresponding to the level of the fourth intercostal space. It is in this formation that open between fifteen and eighteen small orifices that constitute the apertures of the lactiferous ducts. Milk, the stupendous gift of nature for our sustenance, flows therefrom.

There are learned theories to account for the particular disposition of this conspicuous and bilateral, if not wholly symmetrical, organ. And when these schemes refer to evolutionary theory, they invariably present us with a tree-like diagram that shoots forth from a base in which are represented the beings of rudimentary mammary development. Always at the top, as if perched on the crown of a majestic tree, sits the female of the human species, displaying with pride those protrusions that the cantish poetry of the populace has called "twin orbs," "ivory hills," and "orbs of snow." (In what is probably an apocryphal attribution, Alexander Pope is said to have come up, circa 1727, with a gross epithet worthy of a London guttersnipe: "forebuttocks.") The branching lines offer stations for our fellow mammals. Somewhere sits the cat, that has not one, but four on each side, although not all simultaneously active. The two anterior ones, for instance, may be quite dry, leaving the confused kittens of the litter to wrangle among themselves for access to the only active ones. Never at the very bottom of the tree do we find the whale, who has but one pair, yet each measuring six feet in width and one foot in thickness. The lower branches of the schematic tree are reserved for the humble forms of the mammalian class that, bereft of the evolutionary drive toward full differentiation, hardly managed to produce mammary glands: their milk is but a sweaty ooze, that their brood must be content with lapping off the fur of their progenitors. And this, we are reminded, is the pristine fact and substance of all mammary glands, which in spite of their eminence, figurative and literal, are nothing but "modified" sweat glands.

But all the learned theories lack the jolly splendor of Henri de Mondeville's (1260–1320) explanation for the topography of the breasts. In this early surgeon's mind, the matter was quite settled: "The reasons why the breasts of women are on the chest, whereas in other animals they more often appear elsewhere, are of three kinds. Firstly, the chest is a noble, notable, and chaste place. Thus, they can be decently shown. Secondly, warmed by the heart, they return the warmth to it, so that this organ strengthens itself. The third reason applies only to big breasts, which by covering the chest warm, cover, and strengthen the stomach."[2]

It is not the form, but the function of these organs, that bespeaks grandeur. Milk, which is to say life itself, flows abundantly, as from a magic spring. Hardly could we conceive a more direct embodiment of the irrepressible striving of nature. This is why there probably is no more striking representation of a fertility symbol than the Artemis of Ephesus, whose torso is crowded with breasts, like bunched fruits offering themselves to the hunger of our species. When the Goths destroyed her temple in A.D. 262, they found her standing stiffly, as we can see her in the copies of her effigy that survived. All features of the female form have been omitted, as if they were irrelevant. The entire lower part of her body is enclosed in a sort of rigid girdle that tapers towards the feet. She is not the sinuous woman; her lower body is an elongated, inverted cone. And the surface of the column-like ensheathment, divided into compartments, is teeming with reliefs of rams, bees, winged lions, winged bulls, hippogriffs; some of these symbolic animals creep on the forearms of the goddess, the giver of life. Her hands extend outwards, as in a giving gesture. She wears a *modius,* or high-pillared headdress, and behind her head is a disk with more symbolic animals represented on it. The figure is mummy-like, yet we know she is the Great Mother of Life in the exuberant, feracious eclosion of dozens of full, swollen breasts emerging from her torso, just as rows of skulls crowd the chest of Coatlicue, the Aztec Great Mother of Death.

Not in vain did the nomads of Biblical times refer to the paradisiacal land of Palestine as "the land of milk and honey."

For milk is the precious product of millions of years of striving adaptation. It is the one physiologic function that defines us as a class, bestowing upon us the lofty rank that inserts us high in the scale of created beings. For better or for worse, our lot is cast with Mammalia, the class of animals endowed with body hair, small ear bones, ability to stabilize body temperature in a changing environment, and that feature which is at one time badge of strength and source of alienation: a capacious skull containing a well-developed cerebrum. Rightly did we cover lactation with a festoon of emotions. Rightly was milk offered to the prophets, enclosed in leathern bags, to refresh them under the scalding sun of Judea. The Talmud speaks of medicinal properties in goat's milk (B. K. 80a), and a Spanish poet of past centuries, speaking with that passionate accent of his race, not always clear-sighted, pronounced against the custom of surrogate nursing: "Milk is blood/And to nurse your children with someone else's milk/Is like making them bastards."

But between the awesome, seismic commotions that surrounded the development of breasts and the function of lactation, and the aura of triviality that contemporary society spreads over them, what an enormous gap! The organ, viewed in the context of its normal function, is a matter of indifference. Whether to nurse, or not to nurse, is the least of public concerns. An entire generation of Americans was reared with the smell of plastic teats and sterile bottles in lieu of living maternal flesh. And, much in spite of esoteric hypotheses to the contrary, this practice appears not to have had a significant impact on the emotional development of the individuals subject to it. The medical profession cannot be said to have been remiss in its duty to point out the benefits of breast feeding over artificial nursing of infants. The findings are widely publicized: the maternal transfer of antibodies to the infant, via the milk; the protective role of cells passed on to the offspring through this route; or the presence of suspected or definite compounds contained in maternal milk and known to be protective against infections, to which the infant devoid of this defense is susceptible. Thus the medical profession advocates breast feeding as a matter of general principle. General principles, however, are easily overturned by the pressures and demands of society. And in most industrialized societies there has been a powerful drive to modify the recommended practice—namely, the fear of losing the pre-nursing shape of the breast. For in contemporary societies, the female breast has assumed the value of an organ of sexual appeal. And it would be folly, or blindness, to disclaim the immense power of this organ in this regard.

It was not always so. It seems, at least, that in past eras the strength of the breast as a sexual symbol was not the same as today. Scholarly research supports this contention. According to Bruno Roy,[3] a ribald humor anthology of the fifteenth century *(Demandes joyeuses en forme de quolibets)* makes 391 mentions of parts of the human body. As expected in ribald humor, most, or fully 200, refer to the sexual organs (male, 43 percent of the time; female, 57 percent). The breasts, however, are mentioned only four times, and three of these in the context of nursing infants. By the early sixteenth century, however, the quivering of these glandular masses could easily set the whole social fabric atrembling almost anywhere in the civilized world. John Hall, literary figure of the sixteenth century, poetized his righteous indignation in *The Court of Virtue,* where he reminisces,

> *That women theyr breasts did shew and lay out*
> *And well was yt mayd whose dugs then were stoute*
> *Which usance at first came up in the stues*
> *Which mens wyues and daughters after did see.*

"Dugs," he wrote, if there were any doubt that he means invective and ridicule. And by the late sixteenth century breast-related emotions are well polarized in society. Conspicuous display no longer can be carried out with impunity. Thomas Nashe (1567–1601) (toward whom I feel great sympathy for having thought of a title for one of his works that might well have suited the present one: *The Anatomie of Absurditiie*) thundered against the loose mores of his contemporaries. In his work, *Christs Teares over Jerusalem* (1593), he castigates those women who

> *theyr round Roseate buds immodestly lay foorth
> to shew at theyr hands there is fruit to be hoped.*

"Buds" they have now become. And the process of banalization is well under way. The hieratic mystery of lactation is nowhere to be seen. The breast becomes the target for men's fears, desires, doubts, frustrations, and aggressions. The multiplicity of slang and vulgar expressions attests to the complex ambiguity with which it is viewed. Breasts become "hillocks," "butter boxes," and "top ballocks." The popular synonymy goes from the quaintly comical to the fiercely obscene. "Nubbies" used in Australia designates the hallmark of nubility, whereas "boob," according to Webster, is "chiefly Australian" for jail. In America, as we know, the latter word is apt to be taken for a variant of what more discreetly and universally is called "bust." All this is well and good, but "toora-loorals"? The scholarly Peter Fryer,[4] always erudite, informs us that its origin was "theatrical, circa 1909." And we are also told that from the English stage came "langtries," in allusion to the actress Lily Langtry, whom we must suppose a figure of the stage that would be referred to as "full figure" in today's women's magazines. I have heard "lollos," and without claiming credentials in philology (no pun intended) I would be willing to trace the origin of this term to an Italian film star of the not too distant past.

Levity in terminology, however, could not oppose the mighty, invincible magnetic energy irradiating from woman's breasts. "Stronger is their pull than a pair of oxen's on the yoke," says an earthy proverb of the peasants of Jalisco, Mexico. And the prelates of the Church, shuddering at the prodigious force that troubled the peace of their flocks, warned that the laced openings of a woman's bodice were "the gates of hell."[5] Great also were the efforts to close them, including admonitions from the pulpit, and the publication, in the late seventeenth century, of "A Just and Seasonable Reprehension of Naked Breasts and Shoulders," owed to Boileau, historiographer and anti-feminist. All in vain. If, at times, it seemed that the closing of the gates was being achieved, the illusion did not last long. Pious fashion designers endeavored to rebolster what the devil had swung open, but no sooner did they approximate the panels than new doors went ajar at other levels. Modesty along the neckline coincided with exposed shoulders, backs, flanks, or other anatomical regions. Generally, as busts disappeared, legs (a term that couturiers of Victorian times used to designate ankles) appeared.

There is the militant feminist's viewpoint that the whole thing was a Machiavellian male plot to secure women's bondage. The thesis is not without merit. Gordon Rattray Taylor, in a book entitled *The Angel Makers*,[6] comments on the apparent inconsistency of certain fashions in women's apparel that prevailed for some time during the Victorian era. Stays and petticoats (as many as seven petticoats!) were thrown over woman's lower figure, while at the same time the use of low décolletages revealed part of the intermammary cleavage. The idea, in the feminist exegesis, was to suppress the lower part of the female anatomy, being the part viewed as threatening, and to render the woman thus clad utterly sexless. The sole concession was made to the breasts, so that the subject would appear to be Nourisher and Mother, and nothing else. I cannot help but think of the Ephesian Artemis. The goddess was linked to fertility, assisted the women in labor, and presided over wild places as the goddess of vegetation. Yet, she herself was a virgin. The service of her cult, which scholars tell us was orgiastic in nature, was entrusted to mutilated women (amazons) and eunuchs.

Assuming some truth in the charge that males imposed the lowering of the neckline acting on disreputable motives, the result could not have been wider off the mark. For in purposefully unveiling what they had formerly wished to keep covered, they traded places with their prey. Men who were adolescents in the forties still remember the explosive shock to their emerging manhood of the image of the actress Jane Russell recumbent on a haystack, with a daring décolletage, used in the publicity for the otherwise inane film *The Outlaw*. Greater (and presumably healthier) familiarity with the human body than was socially permissible in the forties probably precludes a repetition of the identical phenomenon today. But those who were adolescents then cannot forget the electric jolt that streamed forth from that image. They were sunk into a sort of hypnotic trance, hurled into a precipitous vertical drop, sent gyrating along concentric waves of vertigo, the epicenter of which lay somewhere in that "cleavage," or interhemispherical fissure. Younger generations of men, inured to seeing what their elders veiled with semi-superstitious fear, smile condescendingly at what they deem the ridiculous, outmoded prurience of past ages. But they are unwise to do so. The power in the feminine body is all but eternal. Whether liberally exposed or titillatingly concealed, it emanates vectors of force that are like bridles by which woman sets man's pace, restrains his trot, and governs his every motion.

Women know of this power, and so do men. A college educator who observed the flirting customs of young people was quoted as saying, with a pragmatism that strategists at the Pentagon might have envied: "It is a question not so much of morals as of tactics to consider at what stage in the proceedings they are to be deployed to the best advantage."[7]

Would you stand in awe of the power of a bodily part? Reflect that where there is glory, misery comes not far behind. The law of the body makes no exception of the breast. For in exalting this organ to the state of preponderance and domination that we have described, new forms of slavery sprang forth. Of the new subjections, the first to come is the anxiety that surrounds the normal development of the breasts.

Breast development coincides with the timing of the pubertal growth in height. The breast-bud stage may begin as early as eight years of age, or as late as thirteen: there are early and late "developers." Somewhere between eleven and seventeen years of age, breast development in the female reaches maturity. And what commotions it brings in its wake! The difficult process is not without laughable aspects: the ostentatious affectation of "early developers" who make it known to their classmates in high school that *they* have been the first to join the full ranks of womanhood; the consternation of "late developers" who cower in a corner of the girls' lockers under the gaze of their sniggering, more precocious classmates; and the fulfillment of a modern rite: the first purchase of that form-fitting twin contraption, the "bra," first invented by Monsieur Paul Poiret (1890–1940), to liberate the feminine breast from the armor-like grip of the baleened corset.[8]

Women humorists have described the farcical incidents attending the unfolding of endocrinological physiology. I remember having read an amusing account of a girl's increasing anxiety at the approach of the school prom, in the face of her daily confirmation that what should have been distinctly promontoried remained hopelessly flat. In the last minute, she has resort to "falsies," carefully stuffed with tissue paper. Under the vigorous physical exertion of modern dances, the tissue paper is displaced, producing a peculiar asymmetry for which there is no name in medical treatises, a kind of north-south polarization. She must go back to the ladies' lounge, there to perform the plastic-reconstructive procedure that restores the lost harmony. Tissue paper, alas, becomes friable under conditions of heat and humidity. Much of it has to be sacrificed, else what should be smooth protrusions might look like lumpy gibbosities. As expertly as she can, she manages to perform what in technical parlance could be called a bilateral reduction mammoplasty. Then, she carefully cambers what is left of the original prosthesis, in order to produce a semblance of the initial volume. Her friends call her, the band is playing, and the dance is about to start again. In her youthful enthusiasm to rejoin her companions she runs down the hall, but in turning a corner she hits the recent operative field against an angle of the wall. For the rest of the dance she must display an unbecoming, hollowed-out, one-sided concavity.

The japes of humorists should not hide the more serious aspects of the conflicts that underlie the growth process. One in particular is disturbing, for it seems at the same time normal and pathologic. I refer to the psychologic bestirrings that mammary-gland development invariably elicits.

I must first set down my conviction that the man who tries to understand his own body is doomed to failure. I do not mean this in a purely technical or scientific sense (although here, too, the statement probably applies); rather, I make this affirmation in a sense that might be called, but for the air of pretentiousness that the qualification is bound to bring, philosophical. For understanding is achieved through analysis. The thing examined must be segregated from its surroundings, its parts examined, its components canvassed, and then the object returned to the original context from which it was removed for the purposes of our study. It is because the object interacts with its surroundings that we enrich our study with observations performed after reintegration to the initial context. The method is, therefore, analysis followed by restitution of the object of study to its pristine environment. Most things in the world lend themselves well to this form of study. Not the body. As I type these lines, I am aware that, somehow, I *am* the fingers that type. When I see my friend appear at the door, I am conscious that my friend *is* his bodily structure: tall or short, lean or stout, fair or swarthy. Were he to lose these attributes, I would no longer recognize him. In a sense, he would no longer be himself. In our concept of ourselves, we recognize an absolute correspondence between being and bodily appearance. And two corollaries flow from this. Firstly, that it is impossible to understand our own bodies in a conventional way. For the minute I abstract my body, the moment I study it as an organism, it ceases to be my own self, and becomes a thing. A useful, extraordinary, and necessary instrument, an object of wonder, if you will, but still a thing, and not *me*. Secondly, we recognize that our body, in so far as its coincidence with our being is absolute, is unfelt. At every angle, at every point of their contour, the coincidence between being and body is perfect. And therefore it is unfelt, like a used garment that, from constant use, follows exactly the contour of our silhouette without reminding us of its presence.

Consider now the ominous course of breast development. When the disturbing moment arrives for the child to grow into the woman, the "perfect fit" between body and being is traumatically undone. Whereas the body was formerly unfelt, it is now felt in the mild soreness of the breast buds. And what was formerly taken for granted becomes an object of anxious concern, of fear, sometimes of shame, and always of ambivalence. Even when forewarned by intelligent and sensitive parents, the young girl cannot entirely avoid the anxiety. She surprises men's leers, a chuckle behind her back, an immodest glance. Thus her body, as Simone de Beauvoir so well described in *The Second Sex,* is for the first time "revealed as flesh" to the young girl. And the anxiety brought about by this revelation has well-known effects: she walks with slouching shoulders, and prefers to wear garments that dissimulate the emerging saliences on her chest. But there is no stopping the ineluctable course of life. The world of perfect innocence, of games, the adamantine world of childhood, stays behind. The young girl is now projected forward. To what? The two irrepressible buds on her chest map her future course with implacable accuracy: to sex, to maternity, to the nursing of infants of her own, and then —why not say it?—to death and disintegration.

That most women sort out the entangled web of these conflicts is remarkable in itself. But many are the casualties. For some, the frustration and dissatisfaction with the shape, volume, and the very presence of normal organs reaches heights that men know only when afflicted with serious deformities or conspicuous pathology. It is probably the sense of a threat that leads some of the victims to the hands of the surgeon for deliverance. They expect to be saved—from themselves, from their inability to cope with what society forces them to see as an unsatisfactory bodily image—by the knife of a surgeon.

One of the most beautiful women of whom I have memory was the German wife of an American serviceman. The couple appeared at the emergency room of a hospital where I was an intern, late one night. In the examining room the young woman uncovered the ravishing, supple body of a gazelle, and manually lifted her breasts while looking at me with deep blue eyes in which fear and confusion mingled with a moving plea for help. In the skin of the folds beneath the mammary glands, painful, intensely red and swollen abscessed areas evinced the "pointing" by which the organism manifests that it is about to discharge to the outside the contents of an inflamed tumefaction. Early the next morning, a nurse carried in a basin the two Ivalon sponges that had caused the disorder. These were synthetic prostheses that were then often used, at least in Europe, to artificially enlarge the volume of breasts deemed too small to conform to the majoritarian canons of feminine beauty.

For three decades the incident has not left me. A magnificent body, whose angelic carriage would not have in the least been demerited for want of a few centimeters in chest circumference, had been insensitively tampered with. With her body intact, its bearer would have been no less capable of attracting a mate, and of exercising the whole range of physiologic activities connected with procreation and the nursing of children. Nevertheless she had been sacrificed to the cultural values of the dominant group in the society to which she belonged. And her passivity had allowed her to willingly submit to the bloody rite of contemporary industrial civilizations. The cruel rite through which fears are allayed, dissolved in the total conformity with the norms of the group on physical appearance. Anesthesia, pain, incisions, hospitalizations, and complications: all this she suffered, and more she would have endured, in order to emerge from the rite with a transformed body, a new identity.

Saint Agatha, a Sicilian martyr credited with arresting the eruptions of Mount Etna, suffered the amputation of her breasts, a torture decreed by Quintianus, governor of Sicily, in the year A.D. 251. She appears in her iconography with a sword traversing her breasts, and sometimes carrying her cut-off breasts in a dish.[9] These facts are not irrelevant to my story. I kept a copy of the medical records, and of the histological slides prepared from the tissues of the young German woman. I thought they were an interesting example of the reaction of normal tissue to the presence of foreign material, in this case the prosthesis. By a true coincidence, the report issued by the laboratory states that the day of the operation had been February 5th, the feast of Saint Agatha. And since the day I realized the fortuitous coincidence Saint Agatha ceased to be, for me, the brown virgin of Catania whom the Renaissance masters depict, sadistically handled by cruel centurions who grasp her nipples with forbidding-looking metallic pincers. She is a young *Frau* from Dresden, looking wistfully ahead with eyes of glaucous blue while holding, in a surgical basin, two campanulate, bloodied Ivalon sponges.

But the parade of misery does not end here. The two suns that blazon the glory of woman's attractiveness are also the high sea of woman's suffering. Cancer, the scourge of women in contemporary society, chooses the breast as its preferred site. How to describe the endless succession of extirpated breasts that have come to the laboratory, as the last stage in a worldly career that may once have been glorious? Their once terse and even substance now the seat of inconspicuous indurations or large fungating masses; the once smooth skin now a pitted surface, the *peau d'orange* of clinicians of past ages. And behind each of them a broken life, dashed hopes, tears, and the imminence of an end that appears always too soon, too cruel, and as relentless as it is absurd. No reason to dwell on such misery. Better to shun morbid contemplation, and to cling to today's beliefs: the justified belief that one day this plague will be overcome, and the unjustified belief that with its disappearance there will be no more suffering.

Men in former times, impotent before disease, did not eschew its contemplation. Rather, they surrounded our ills with stories and legends, as a means of asking forbearance from overwhelming calamity. I should like to end with one of them, because it is one that places the female breast in curious apposition with the life of a mystic. The man was Raymond Llull, one of the most intriguing minds of the Middle Ages.[10]

In Raymond Llull (1235–1316) nature produced an extraordinary combination: the contemplative and the man of action. It is fitting that such a reaction product should crystallize only rarely in nature's alembics. For the potential energy of the synthesis puts the universal equilibrium in jeopardy. The son of one of the gallant knights that followed King Don Jaime in his campaigns for the conquest of the Balearic Islands, Llull was reared at the court of Majorca. From the Moors there he learned Arabic, and later founded colleges where missionaries were taught semitic languages before leaving to convert the Saracens to Christianity. We see him now leading the life of an anchorite and receiving mystical visions, now preaching in Syria, Palestine, and Ethiopia, where he endures the mockeries of heathens who "gave him blows and pulled at his beard." Then he is back again in Europe, teaching his personal brand of Neoplatonism in Montpellier, or debating the Averroists in Paris. And this indefatigable theologian, mystic, and poet still found time to write over five hundred books, some in prose, some in verse, some in Latin, and some in his native Catalan, the structural bases of which he helped to lay down.

This whirlwind of activity is not enough to content him. He must sail to Bougie, in North Africa, where he is sure to persuade the Muslims to acknowledge the fallacy of their creed. He sails from Palma on August 14, 1316, and barely disembarked he challenges fifty Arab doctors to public debate on the very beach of his landing. The zeal of his mission, however, blinds him to the dangers of fanaticism. Too vivid a figure of speech, or a peroration too emphatic; who knows? The fact is that in his transports of eloquence he fails to detect the anger in the eyes of his listeners, outraged at the effrontery of an infidel who mocks the sacred truths of Islam in the land of its prophet. "Death to the infidel!" sounds one. And this exhortation is followed by a savage rain of stones hurled at the venerable figure of the preacher. A large rock cracks his skull, and fragments of the softish grey matter that conceived the *Ars Magna* roll on the ground, caked with sand. The rib cage that encloses a heart still incandescent with the love of God is furiously kicked by the mob until its last glow dies out. When the crowd disperses, Genoese merchants approach the deserted beach, pick up the limp, lifeless body, wash the gore off the white beard and the ragged frock, and transport the mortal remains of Llull back to Majorca.

It was not long before miracles were said to be occurring at the tomb of the martyr. The church welcomed the veneration of the man who so fervidly, if tactlessly, had toiled in its service. But it moved slowly, as always, in pronouncing itself on the question of sainthood. Under Popes Clement XIII and Pius VI, his veneration was approved. Under Pius IX, Llull received the designation of *Beato* (Blessed), a station on the road to full sainthood, implying only limited public religious honors.

If we search for the springs that impelled this extraordinary man to his achievements, we find a curious episode. It seems that he was not always the beatific soul of his later years. Like Francis of Assisi, or Augustine of Hippo, he passed his youth in thrall to the vanities and pleasures that he later condemned. The chivalric customs of the court of Majorca were good training to render a young man sensitive to feminine charms. Llull showed himself here, too, a discerning pupil. He succumbed to the attraction of Ambrosia del Castello, a Genoese beauty residing in Majorca. Mad with desire, he pursued the woman with the obsessive intensity that characterized all his projects. It seems that he was married already. This did not impede him from pressing the chase beyond the bounds that his contemporaries set to social decorum. The Majorcan tradition has it that, one day, he wooed the belle while he straddled his steed, as the lady hurried on down the street to avoid public embarrassment.

Undaunted by her efforts to avoid him, he followed her through narrow streets and into the central plaza of the town. And when she slipped into the church, the bold pursuer entered the sacred precinct on horseback. Tradition says that this has been the only time that the sound of horse's hooves reverberated under the ancient vitrailed windows of Saint Eulalia's temple, distracting the shocked faithful from the holy rites of Mass.

A passion that thought little of outraging the pious, however, balked at a single gesture of the woman so ardently coveted. When at last he contrived to accost her in a solitary place, and expressed to her the perfervid desire that consumed him, she drew him aside, loosened the ties of her bodice, opened her undergarments, and exposed to the sedulous pursuer a breast half devoured by an ulcerated cancer. Shaken by this experience, Llull thought no more of the vain and frivolous concerns of his youth. He took up the monk's coarse cloth, left behind family and friends, and set out on the road where he descried, coruscating and distant, the crown of martyrdom.[10]

The Anorectum

The intestine is a long and flexuous tube; it moves with sluggish contractions that spread like waves, rippling downwards. Its function is double: to retain and to expel. Thus, its wisdom vastly surpasses the niggardly estimates made of it: it must discern what is useful and what is waste. Ultimately the sole concern of intelligence is to distinguish between grain and chaff. It is no small irony that this discrimination is entrusted both to the most valued and the most disdained of our parts. Yet greater irony lies in the fact that, when it comes to competence and trustworthiness, the scale weighs heavily on the side of the most disdained.

The ascertainment is carried out through an ingenious specialization of structure. Where food digestion and absorption predominate, the intestinal tube is narrow and coiled; where residues solidify and are readied, so to speak, for expulsion, the tube becomes widened. In herbivorous animals this wide tube, known as the large intestine, is longer than in carnivores. Man is an omnivorous creature, but his spiritual affiliation is with the carnivores, and he breeds true in matters colonic: his colon measures between 91 and 125 centimeters, which is distinctly short (by reference to ratios of nose-anus length to body length).[1] Thus man may be said to be in harmony with his kind, the carnivores. The large intestine describes the looped course that schoolboys learn to recite. It ascends, crosses over, descends, twists like an *S*, and finally, at the level of the third or fourth sacral vertebra, it becomes a somewhat ampullar bag. Here, its inner lining loses its formerly corrugated appearance, and the tube zigzags its way toward the anal canal. The name for this sinuous last portion of the large bowel makes sense only to those attuned to anatomical nomenclature. It is called the *rectum,* from the Latin word meaning "straight."

What first strikes the student is that he has come across a repository of filth. He may wonder at the existence of shelf-like folds, the *valves of Houston,* denting the lumen of the rectum, and at the exquisite structural refinement that dots the rectal lining with myriads of tiny pits into which open the remarkable *glands of Lieberkühn.* But before these marvels are revealed, feces must be set aside, the stench of refuse must be endured. The price is here exacted in fortitude and resignation. It was paid by Houston, and in the same coin by Lieberkühn; lesser men will not be exempted. The rectum is a paradoxical organ. For the first thought that it evokes is inevitably a second-order idea, wrung out of hurt sensibilities: why should the body resort to such offensive concentration, when excreta could be gently vaporized, eliminated molecule by molecule, insensibly. Elsewhere shines the grandeur of the body while its misery, concealed, lurks behind. But here beauty hides behind misery concretized and obtrusive. Nowhere is the essential antinomy of our nature better symbolized.

Moralists used the contradiction well. The effectiveness of their rhetoric was much enhanced by its use. In one of his homilies, Chrysostom describes a splendid banquet: the birds from Phasis, the soups mixed with multiple ingredients, the delicate meats roasted on embers. "Burst now in thought the belly of them who feed on such things, and thou wilt see the vast refuse, the unclean channel, and the whited sepulchre. . . ." For such is the unavoidable end of our pleasures, the fundamental limitation inherent in our bodies. Will you feed on dainties, and gorge yourself with elaborate delicacies, the exquisitely refined dishes that tempt the eye and the palate? Be reminded that "what come after these, I am ashamed to tell, [are] the disagreeable eructations, the vomitings, the discharges downwards and upwards. . . ." The ascetics' only countermeasure is fasting. Since bestiality and corruption reside in our nature, at least let the feed be restricted that invigorates the beast and promotes its putrefaction. "Stand nigh the man who fasts and thou wilt straightaway partake of his good odor; for fasting is a spiritual perfume; and through the eyes, the tongue, and every part, it manifests the good disposition of the soul."[2] Thus, the mystic condemns organic decomposition because he condemns the site in which it occurs: the body of a man.

But we are not mystics. Try as we may, our corporeal nature keeps weighing us down. Useless to dwell on the ingeniousness of our design, or on the semi-ethereal nature of our recondite chemistry: we are not disembodied spirits. Our body is at one time airy and substantial; and in the plan of superior harmony that one day must reign, room must be made to accommodate the anorectum. We hardly need psychologists to remind us that every human being must pass through a pregenital, anal phase of development. It is a fact of daily observation that the lot of man is closely tied up with the manner in which he comes to terms with his anorectum. The prim, the perfectionist, and the maudlin live in perpetual disgust. And this conflict manifests itself in spasm, constipation, and an extraordinary obsession with subduing a rebellious, self-willed bowel. Or anxiety may take the form of the so-called "irritable bowel syndrome," in which nervous discharges are mirrored in what Saint Chrysostom dubbed the "downward discharges." The syndrome is currently ill-defined. But wherever its true boundaries may lie, its hallmark is exaggerated rectal responsiveness to emotion. Which suggests that the "mirror of the soul" may actually reside on an anatomical plane lower than poets have surmised.

Individuality stamped in rectal discharges is today a frivolous idea. It was not always so, if one considers the practices of ancient physicians and divinators, who read man's destiny and personality in his dejections. And there is no denying that the idea may one day become again creditable. In *The Rebel Angels,* the delightful, festive novel by the Canadian writer Robertson Davies, a doctoral student in the humanities visits a scientist whose field of specialization is human feces. After being shown more about the structure and composition of human refuse than most people care to know, the humanist muses on how past ages, living closer to the world of nature, expressed in their language a lively concern for all that relates to the body, not excluding the disagreeable excrementitious residues that our modern antiseptic era peremptorily blots out of consciousness. Thus, the Middle Ages had specific terms for the feces of different animals: "the Crotels of a Hare, the Friants of a Boar, the Spraints of an Otter, the Werderobe of a Badger, the Waggying of a Fox, the Fumets of a Deer." And what has our time to oppose to this acutely discriminating lexicon? A single word, four-lettered, that Webster says is "usu. considered vulgar." This ignominious verbal indigence cannot be tolerated by Robertson Davies's fictional humanist, who takes up the challenge with the gusty positiveness of a vindicator, and suggests a contemporary terminology: Why not "the Problems of a President, the Backward Passes of a Footballer, the Deferrals of a Dean, the Odd Volumes of a Librarian, the Footnotes of a Ph.D., the Low Grades of a Freshman, the Anxieties of an Untenured Professor?"[3]

Aside from whimsical references of this kind, the anorectum and its contents, whose very existence is obstinately denied by the modern mind, long found no place in literature. It is perhaps no coincidence that the Spanish soul, at one and the same time earthy and mystic, managed to smuggle this anatomic substratum into the world of letters. Don Francisco de Quevedo y Villegas (1580–1645), the most complex personality of Spain's "Golden Century," managed to write both sublime treatises on theological questions and vitriolic satires on the follies of his time.[4] He may be thought of as a sort of revised and augmented version of Swift. Schoolteachers in the Spanish-speaking world shudder to assign works of this master satirist to their pupils; not all should be read by young minds, for Quevedo could be facetious, mocking, or unmitigatedly obscene. One of his early works, written in 1620 and published in 1626, is entitled *Graces and Disgraces of the Eye of the Ass.* Once and for all, the anorectum acceded to Parnassus, by the hand of a truly great poet and satirist; and all men of letters since, if they are to frequent Parnassus, must be, to some degree, proctologists.

The Eye of the Ass is here presented as more praiseworthy than the eyes of the face. "Its place is median, like that of the sun; its feel is soft; it has but one eye, and because of this some have wished to disparage it, calling it one-eyed. But in truth this is also praiseworthy, for so it comes to resemble the Cyclopes, who themselves were one-eyed and descended from the gods of sight." And later we are edified by learning of its most noble history and innocent character, for some "anchorites, to remain chaste, plucked out the eyes of the face, which the saints and good Christians called windows of the soul. Because of them we have lovesickness, rape, adultery, deaths, rage, and theft. But when did the peaceable and virtuous Eye of the Ass cause a scandal in the world, restlessness, or war?" Moreover, the eyes of the face are dispensable, in addition to being potentially nefarious. Not so the "middle eye," which besides being always excellent, is absolutely indispensable to the continuance of life.

Having covered the "graces," our satirist turns his attention to the "disgraces," or misfortunes, of the organ object of his labors. He lists seventeen "disgraces." All are instances in which, by his own observation, the fundament is maligned. For instance, the third one: "Come the slouch and the miserable cadger, who, eager to fill their stomachs for free, stuff themselves beyond measure; and it is the ass who pays a high price for the indulgence, exacted by the nuzzle of the [enema's] fountain-syringe." To summarize, which is what Quevedo purports to do in the seventeenth "disgrace," such is the ill star of this organ that it finds punishment even in the very exercise of its normal function. "All bodily parts delight in what they do: the eyes of the face in contemplating beauty; the nose, in aspiring pleasant odors; the mouth, in tasting seasonings and viands; and the tongue frolicking in laughter and chatter. But, once that the ass wished to please itself, it got singed."

Now with all due respect to the egregious figure of Quevedo, I must say that in this little work of his I see much that is vulgar banality, with limited relevance for the modern reader. To be sure, there is an unexampled virtuosity in the use of the language, and such forceful, scalding satirical style as one would look for in vain in his contemporaries (in or out of Spain), or in ours. Quevedo yields to no one in his power of unleashing bitter irony with colorful realism. But apart from the genial stylistic imprint of its author, *Graces and Disgraces* is marred by an excessive propensity toward the gross pun, the untranslatable conundrum or baroque conceit, and, all too often, the crassitude of a past era less than keen to adhere to principles of hygiene that, to our great fortune, have become part of modern culture. Nevertheless, the work remains today an interesting document. Not so much on account of its ideas (which I find often reducible to the youthful gropings of its author in that miry zone of the Spanish baroque that was later called *conceptismo*), as due to the mysterious springs from where it may have originated. Admittedly, the origins of a work of art are never clear. But it is a safe assumption that maintains that all circumstances surrounding the life of its author converge, like tributary rivulets, into the copious stream. And the life circumstances of Quevedo could hardly have been more striking.

Consider the times of our man. In the seventeenth century, artistic forms abandoned the Renaissance models. The idealized conceptions yielded to the new reality, astir with political, social, and all sorts of unrest. In Spain, where traditionally contrasts have tended to reach unwholesome tensions, this new reality was especially tangible. The hallucinating gold of the New World arrived daily in massive cargoes, then vanished the next day without causing benefit to the needy, or satiety to the venal men in power. Philip II died saying with regret that God, who gave him so many kingdoms, had denied him a son capable of ruling them. Our author was then eighteen years of age, and dreamed of a political career. The King's successor saw fit to transfer the court to Madrid in 1606, and the capital of the kingdom became the meeting place for job-seekers, parvenus, favorites, and parasites of every conceivable description.

Opportunism, greed, rampant illegality, and corruption soon degraded an aristocracy never known for equanimity or temperance. The nerve and sinew of the nation, the proud hidalgo, on whose shoulders Spain had been lifted to the place of highest preeminence in Europe (and therefore in the world), followed suit in the moral disintegration, or was absorbed into an underworld of *pícaros*, there to lead a difficult, hand-to-mouth existence in discouragement or cynicism. The fields deserted, the people starving, and the once awesome empire locked in irreversible decline, there was little left to a man of Quevedo's mold but to inveigh against those ills, in tones ever more poisoning and indignant. Does all this have anything to do with his writing the *Graces and Disgraces?* More, perhaps, than appears at first sight. He observed a decomposing society. And when the ideas of decomposition, filth, putrefaction, and decay are once present to the mind, the possible surging associations are infinite. However, the idea of excreta most insistently insinuates itself, in either the superficial or deep strata of the mind, because it is one that is reiterated in the daily activities of the body.

And let us note that the idea of riches is also not too far away. Gold as excrement is an old metaphor that has thrived ubiquitous in the mind of poets, or of the disaffected and impractical (which is really saying the same thing). Gold is wrested out of "the bowels of the earth," and our lives pass by constantly under its dominating sign, independently of our sentiments on the matter. The parallel extends further. There is something repugnant in the tendency to hoard it; its normal fate ought to be expulsion and dispersal, for only thus can it reveal the life-giving, fertilizing properties that hide in it. The roots of Quevedo's scatological turn of mind are thus not difficult to trace to this vision of a lifeless metal worsening the lives of his compatriots as it arrived in the galleons that sailed up the Guadalquivir from the colonies. The Mexican poet Octavio Paz[5] quotes Marx as having tried to define the conditions that prevail in capitalist society with this aphorism: "the domination of living men by dead matter." But Paz adds that a more precise formulation would have been obliged to qualify the statement by saying that it is a "domination by *abstract* dead matter," since today it is not material gold, as in Quevedo's Spain, that asphyxiates us, but rather a whole symbolic network of credit cards, banknotes, stocks, and bonds that has taken the place of gold ingots and silver bars to oppress us. New alchemy of our age: the transmutation of excrement into certificates of deposit. An achievement undreamt of by even the most credulous searchers of the philosophical stone.

I will not go so far as to discuss the theories of psychiatrists who have seen a relationship between anal eroticism and capitalism. There is here a fertile imagery. If the child naturally plays with his feces, why would the child in the grown man not prolong the game with a fecal equivalent? And is there not a connection between anal retention and a preponderant impulse to economize, to regulate wisely what is spent, and to limit waste? What if a connection were discovered between theories on economics and the bowel habits of the theoreticians? Some, like the poet Octavio Paz, have exploited the "excremental vision of the world" to limits that baffle more pedestrian imaginations. Trained in the habit that refuses to confer to bodily functions meanings other than the strictly clinical and physiological, my mind stubbornly refuses to soar aloft in the company of such visionaries. I seriously doubt that the Calvinist ethic stems from a desire to counteract an impulse to excremental waste and dispersal; nor can I give much credence to notions that say that restrictive theologies arise from a need to "deodorize" and sublimate the inevitable putrefactions in the normal cycle of life. But clinical observation is sufficient to convince me that the anorectum—"end of terminus," as Quevedo called it— is some kind of mysterious avatar of the grandeur and misery of the body. With emphasis, it seems, on the misery.

Some learn to live with it. Others find the mere thought insufferable and pretend it does not exist. Still others subject themselves to the rigors of conscious denial. The comical scientist in Robertson Davies's novel explored human typology through human excreta. The question is more serious than this humoresque jab would suggest. Endomorphs and ectomorphs are very real human types; their respective preoccupations will keep alive the controversy of nature versus nurture for a long time to come. Take one type. Call it, for brevity, type A: as thin as a whisper or an exhalation, stretched like the apostles of El Greco, seemingly uncomfortable in this temporary bodily encasement that it seems always on the verge of quitting, from above. Contrast it to its opposite, which we all know but dare not call a distinct type. Call it type B, for convenience: wide, rotund, expanded, as if pulled down, offering all its mass to the gravitational pull. The former would suppress the rectal function, if it were in his power, and reacts usually with the spastic tonicity of denial to the pressures of the world. This one, the type B, is all acceptance and earthiness, and finds nothing easier in his constitution than "to bear down" when required. If they exist at all, these two types represent idealized extremes; they are "archetypes." But the temptation is great to assign most human beings to a position in this schematic scale, and to draw the conclusions that this fanciful construct anticipates.

In one case, denial of a natural physiologic function is believed to maim the personality: the type A human being lives in perpetual danger of this excess. It is not difficult to find upholders of this opinion. The theory that too severe toilet training during early childhood wreaks havoc in the mind is now part of the popular lore. A few years ago an Englishman, Ian Gibson, defended this very thesis in a book entitled *The English Vice.* [6] This author attempted to show that a streak of sadism has run deep in English society since Victorian times, manifested in a proclivity to administer whippings to children, in and out of school; a sadistic coloring was also perceived in other spheres of English life. It was contended that, compared to Southern European countries in which defecation is not an unmentionable act, the English fare poorly on the humanitarian social scale. I need not mention the massive professional literature that purports to link these observations as cause and effect. No doubt Ian Gibson drew heavily from those sources to strengthen his arguments. I leave it to professionals in the behavioral sciences to determine the validity of his thesis. On the other hand, too emphatic an acceptance of anorectal functions could be, if not as damaging, at least equally unseemly. Recall Rabelais, the epitome of what has been called here, quite arbitrarily, a type B. And see him writing a full-length book chapter on rump-wiping (the famous chapter of the first book of the life of Gargantua, that some English translators—type A people, no doubt—refused to translate), or rather, on the invention of the perfect rump-wiper by a child prodigy. Ends the Gargantuan peroration: "In conclusion, I will state and maintain that there is no rump-wiper like a good downy goose, providing that you hold its head between your legs. . . . And do not think that the beatitude of the heroes and demigods in the Elysian Fields comes from their asphodel, or their ambrosia, or their nectar. Those are old wives' tales. In my humble opinion, it comes from the fact that they wipe their arses with the neck of a goose. And such, also, is the opinion of Master John of Scotland."

Like the translator who "recoiled" from rendering that chapter into English, I, too, had strong reservations about narrating another unbecoming excess of the type B faction. How to describe examples of bad taste without incurring the charge of bad taste ourselves? In deference to the reader, I here protest of my initial intention to omit altogether the anecdote that follows. These scruples vanished, however, when I found out that an Italian film was recently exhibited in the United States that traced the biography of the singular personage who is the chief protagonist of the story. No reason to be secretive about it any more: the facts are, as they say, in the public domain. The film—and the *nom de guerre* of our man—was *Il Petomano*. To my recollection, no translation was offered for this film in America. I suppose "The Wind-Breaker" would have been an accurate translation, although perhaps not the film title most apt to attract a very large public.

Sarah Bernhardt was packing the largest theater in Paris, and without fail moving her audience to tears with her art, when "Il Petomano," gifted with an altogether different sort of artistry, was hired to perform at the *Moulin Rouge*. Ziedler, the impresario, received the uncommon "virtuoso" one afternoon, after having been told by his assistants that he ought to see this man, "a real phenomenon," sure to astonish the clientele with his uncanny talent. The interview has been set down in print by Marcel Pagnol, who heard all about it from Yvette Guilbert, who in turn was present at the event and knew its main *dramatis personae*. I here follow Pagnol's account.[7]

Less than eager, Ziedler agreed to receive the tall, austere visitor:

"I understand, Monsieur," said Ziedler, "that you have an uncommon ability. May we know what it is?"

"Quite so, Monsieur," explained the visitor with an air of utter seriousness. "You see, I have what you might call a vacuum-aspirator anus."

Ziedler, used to unconventional characters in show business, sounded somewhat diffident when he said, jokingly:

"Really? Good for you!"

The visitor, unperturbed and with a pedantic air, went on:

"You see, thanks to a system of muscular discipline of my own devising, I have achieved an extraordinary control. Something beyond the reach of most human beings. Something, to my knowledge, never before attempted."

"No kidding! What, if we may know, can you do?"

"I can, for example, aspirate a not inconsiderable amount of fluid."

"You mean you can actually drink from behind? This I have to see! And what shall I offer you?"

"Bring me a large pail of water, or a filled wash basin."

"Straight away. Mineral water, or plain? What is your pleasure, Monsieur?"

"I will take plain, Monsieur, thank you."

The water basin was brought in, and our man, having untied a special aperture in his performing costume, sat on it and proceeded to carry out the feat he had announced. After a few minutes, he disclosed with the same pedantic air that he was going to revert the process, and returned the "ingested" fluid to the original container. At the completion of the act, a certain sulphurous odor diffused through the room.

"Amazing! You can also elaborate Enghien water!" said Ziedler, alluding to a site known for its sulphurous, presumably medicinal waters.

"Wrong," replied his interlocutor without flinching. "This I call my preparatory rinsing. Having performed this . . . er . . . internal ablution, I am ready to go on with my act, which consists in the emission of sounds from the anorectal canal, but so controlled in pitch by the action of the sphincterian muscles, that . . ."

"You mean you are now going to fart?"

"Monsieur! If you please! What I mean is that I can produce at will a variety of sound pitches."

"I am overwhelmed!" exclaimed Ziedler. And he proceeded to listen to a veritable recital of posteriorly generated sounds, ranging from basso profundo to coloratura soprano, the whole achieved through physical principles governing the passage of air currents through a sound instrument of deftly controlled diameter, and at equally well-controlled flow rates.

The man was signed up on the spot.

What the end was of this singular artist, I have no idea. But what is generally known, since it has become part of the history of the famed Parisian show-business extravaganzas of the early part of this century, is that the publicity for his act was adver-

tised on a large affiche at the door of the Moulin Rouge that
read:

WILL PERFORM TODAY
FROM 9 TO 9:30 P.M.
IL PETOMANO
THE ONLY ARTIST WHO IS UNAFRAID OF
COPYRIGHT INFRINGEMENTS

The Body and
the Emotions

In what follows I am to describe the emotions—what past and pithier ages called the passions—knowing full well the futility of my task. For it is obvious that these mental states are barely known, not yet counted, described in the sketchiest manner, and understood not at all. Spinoza reduced their mickle number to three: joy, sadness and desire, but one may suspect this to be a gross underestimate, when one considers their virtually endless subspecies and combinations. For the emotions are not static and immutable, but in perpetual flux, forever giving rise to new and hybrid entities. So that the emotional fauna and flora that result are of such complexity that the immense diversity of the natural world pales by comparison. Ortega y Gasset once wrote that botanists and zoologists have been left free to classify living beings into millions of species (and their catalog is probably still incomplete), without anyone taking the trouble to accuse them of "Byzantinism." Psychologists deal with a world as rich in classifiable entities as that of biologists, but seem content to use a crude and most rudimentary classification in what is, to all appearances, a field of mind-boggling intricacy.

The warp and woof of the emotions has heretofore been described from two main vantage points: from the psychology laboratories, or from the armchair of philosophers. In the first case, what is delivered to us is nothing but the skin, as it were, the superficial layers of the specimen we would like to dissect. In the second case, we must be content with dissecting shadows. For if there is an interpretation that transcends the outward appearance of the emotions, it must be one that lays bare our innermost nature, and addresses such questions as the origin of our conduct in the world, the forces that control our acts, and the scope and limits of our perfectibility. In other words, it must belong in metaphysics, that branch of knowledge that was most ably defined by D'Alembert's housekeeper as "the investigation of what any man of common sense already knows, or of what no man will ever know, and, in either case, a perfectly useless knowledge."

ON LAUGHTER

The Greeks assigned an internal seat to hilarity: the diaphragm. From its contractions issues laughter that is utterly corporeal, not born of passion; hence the laughter provoked by nudges in the ribs, which is where the diaphragm inserts. The warlike customs of the ancient Romans added one more curious observation, that gladiators laughed upon receiving wounds on their flanks. "Does it hurt? Only when I laugh," is a piece of wry humor older than usually surmised: it was probably first heard on the steps of the Colosseum. Juan Luis Vives, Spanish scholar and disciple of Erasmus, explained the uncontrollable laughter that seizes those deprived of food for a long time, when at last they are able to partake of a meal. The reason is the excitation of the diaphragm that, wrinkled, contracted and grown stiff, at last suddenly distends and relaxes.[1] I suspect the spare life style of a sixteenth-century scholar furnished Vives more than one occasion to observe this pathetic phenomenon directly in his own person. But he does not belabor this observation. His main concern is to warn us that there are real and inauthentic forms of laughter. Thus, when sadness and indignation prevail, laughter is suspect. Hannibal was said to laugh in the Carthaginian Senate after his defeat by the Romans, but, says Vives, it appears more likely that faulty observers may have mistaken teeth-grinding for laughter.

There is assuredly something mechanical in laughter, since it can be provoked by tickling the armpits, the soles, the groin, or the abdomen. It all begins in the face: the corners of the mouth are pulled back and elevated; the upper lip tenses and the teeth are exposed; the cheeks seem puffed up and pushed against the lower eyelids; the eyes are partly closed and shining. Then, there is a strange vocalization: air is deeply inspired, and then expelled with short, spasmodic contractions that physiologists term "inspiration-expiration microcycles."[2] When its intensity increases, the whole body seems convulsed, and respiration is greatly disturbed. Have you ever mistaken the man who sobs for the man who laughs, or the man who laughs for the one who sobs? I have, and do not believe that this mistake is to be wondered at, since the appearance of the two is so greatly similar: in both there may be a strange change of sound, as if the larynx vibrated during a deep inspiration, which is then followed by short, saccadic, spastic motions. In both the face is flushed, and, most remarkable of all, in both tears may roll. And yet it is plain that the winds that agitate the one are blowing in a direction precisely opposite to that of the gales that shake the other.

In laughter, the direction of this movement is thought to be upwards. It is a tendency of our whole being toward buoyancy, a force that uplifts, a magnet that polarizes all life processes to the positive side. Not only metaphorically, but in a real sense, with a reality that may be objectively tested in measurements of our bodily chemistry. Norman Cousins has told us of his victory over ankylosing spondylitis, a disease for which no definitive cure is yet available, by a regimen that included heavy doses of hilarity. Where others submit to periodic injections, steroids, and analgesics, Cousins had his nurse read to him jokes out of humor anthologies at fixed intervals; films of jocular nature were projected on a screen placed in front of his sickbed.

These were essential, and in his view decisive, components of his therapy. Faced with this continuous barrage of laughs, the subcutaneous nodules receded, the stiffness of the joints abated, the pain gradually diminished, and the erythrocyte sedimentation rate returned to normal levels.[3]

The broad-minded physician is not ashamed to admit that he believes in the possibility of writing, in the future, a medical prescription that might read as follows:

R̟

Sardonic Tittering
Every 4 hours

Loud Guffaws
One before each meal

Silly Giggles
Quantum sufficit.

One problem stands in the way, however. If laughter is to be beneficial, it must itself be "healthy." For there are several kinds of laughter: there is one that is embittered, and one that springs from pain, and one that acknowledges our unresolved conflicts. And there is also a form that is wholly pathologic. It may be the equivalent of an epileptic fit: some patients have been known to laugh uncontrollably when prey to the disordered, chaotic bursts of nervous energy that characterize epilepsy ("gelastic seizure").[4] There are clinical descriptions of patients affected by tumors of the brain, in whom laughter appeared every time the patient purposefully directed his gaze to one side (saccadic lateral eye movements did not produce the same effect), and was no longer observed after the tumor was removed by the neurosurgeon.[5] In other cases, hyperventilation, or an exaggerated extension of the back, sufficed to bring about uncontrollable fits of laughter. Pathological laughter may be accompanied by a true feeling of hilarity, if the reports of the patients themselves are to be considered trustworthy. Like pestilence, this laughter may spread. In East Africa hysterical laughter afflicted almost one thousand persons between 1962 and 1964, predominantly girls: schools were closed, parents of victims of the laughing epidemic suffered contagion, and the disease spread to neighboring villages; exhausted by laughter, some patients required hospitalization.[6] Of these unfortunates it may be said that they were unhappy because they laughed, and happy when they ceased to laugh. And it would not increase our accuracy to say that they substituted one kind of laughter for another one, since we do not know how to define the one any better than the other. Hence the physician, who does not presume to measure what he does not understand, must remain content with concluding that he has witnessed this paradoxic exception to the law that rules human affairs: that his patient was getting better *because* he laughed less.

It follows that the foremost concern of our future therapist should be a careful canvassing of the forms of laughter, since only some, but not all, have healing properties. And so, we witness this extraordinary phenomenon (which, however, is not entirely without precedent), that the investigation of the causes of hilarity, heretofore left in the hands of metaphysicians, becomes the rightful province of medical men. They must strive to tell us where are the springs of hilarity, where lies true laughter, the real, spontaneous, life-giving laughter.

What others have said cannot be ignored, even if their statements fail to satisfy our curiosity.[7] Kant, I am afraid, would have voted for the abolition of all emotions, which he regarded as illnesses of the mind; laughter, accordingly, would have been the mere symptom of an ailment, though one trivial and inconsequential, when compared to the malignancy of other "passions." And the emphasis on the meaninglessness of the symptom is further assurance that Kant is not worried over the prognosis, for to him laughter arises when one realizes that there is nothing where something was expected—"the sudden transformation of a strained expectation into nothingness."

To believe Bergson, laughter implies a certain psychic an-

kylosis, a sort of stiffness of the soul, since it shoots forth automatically, before reflection. Moreover, it is the essence of the
comic to manifest as robot-like automatism. In the Bergsonian
formula, the clown who receives a pie in the face is comic on
account of his rigidity: he should have ducked, thereby avoiding
the missile. Instead, he remained rigid, uncompliant, the target
of pie-throwing, or bastinades, or any of the numerous insults
known for their effectiveness in producing laughter in slapstick
comedy. Couples who dance seem "funny" if one abstracts the
music, because then they resemble mannekins. The actor in a
comedy who recites lines out of tempo is invariably laughable.
Comedy writers profit from this circumstance. Imagine the de-
livery of a congratulatory speech to a man who did not win the
lottery, but, instead, lost his fortune. Or, condolences offered to
the relatives of a survivor. The speech might have been appropriate at one time, perhaps two or three scenes before in the
comedy, but circumstances have now changed. The comedian
should have modified his speech to suit the new conditions, but
persists in his formerly chosen course out of rigidity. And it is
this rigid momentum, this automatism, which in Bergson's
scheme accounts for the effect of being "funny."

I always professed great admiration for this theory of the
nature of the comic. It seemed to me that Bergson had, if nothing else, shown himself as supremely clever. For it was difficult
to conceive of comical situations which could not be "explained," more or less directly, by this formula. I was therefore
somewhat disturbed to see an altogether different interpretation of these facts, admirably expounded by Marcel Pagnol, the
playwright.[8] We laugh, he said, not because the comic is rigid,
but because we feel ourselves superior to those locked in its
rigidity. This theory is, of course, neither new nor Pagnol's. It
is already mentioned by Thomas Hobbes, who was born in the
sixteenth century (prematurely, it seems, when his mother
delivered before her expected date of confinement out of fear
of the approaching Spanish Armada), and he probably took it
from Greco-Roman antiquity. It may be called the theory of

"sudden glory," for Hobbes stated (*Human Nature*, ch. IX) that laughter comes from "sudden glory arising from the sudden conception of some eminence in ourselves, by comparison with the infirmity of others, or with our own formerly." However, I prefer Marcel Pagnol's exposition. Having written some of the funniest comedy scenes for the contemporary stage, he has as much right to be heeded on the subject of what makes people laugh, as the most ponderous philosopher. He has made me laugh, and kept me attentive and excited, which is more than I can say for Hobbes, I must admit.

Imagine a scene in which an actor is going to punish an affront by delivering a sonorous kick on the offender's backside, or another scene in which he is about to declaim an amorous speech to his mistress. The comedy writer could contrive, in the first instance, a set of circumstances whereby a haughty and feared personage—say, the actor's boss in the play—puts on the clothes of the intended victim, and is sighted by the aggressor from behind. The comic effect would be greatly enhanced by the preparations with which the kicker, facing the public, relishes the imminence of his revenge. Likewise, in the second example, the playwright could create a scene in which the wife replaces the mistress just before the appearance of the actor representing the philanderer. The comic effect would benefit from this substitution remaining unknown to the unfaithful man for some time, so that he might address the wife as if she were the mistress, to the merriment of the theater's audience. But these typical scenes of farce are interpreted in radically different ways by the theoreticians of humor. Bergson would have us believe that discernment of the rigidity of the comedian's actions is sufficient cause to make us laugh: the kicker's behavior persisting unaltered, or the philanderer's conduct remaining unchanged, in spite of the change of the circumstances that prompted their respective acts. Pagnol, the "tastiest" expositor of the theory of "sudden glory," attaches a moral significance (and one not exactly flattering to our nature) to our laughter. We laugh out of uncharitableness, because we experience our superiority with respect to the clown. He proceeds to kick his boss's behind, but *we* would never make such a gross mistake. He addresses the wife with the words that he had prepared for the mistress, but if ever *we* found ourselves in that predicament, *we* would unfailingly discover the trap, and would pull ourselves out of trouble with as much grace and agility as a ballet dancer executing a perfectly timed step. Laughter is made the cognate of arrogance.

Could it be that there is something blamable, something reprehensible at the origin of all laughter? What if we were to find a streak of the malevolent, or of the unpitying, hiding behind all forms of laughter, including those that we believe most "wholesome"? This would be a shocking discovery, for then the physician would become at one and the same time the advocate of the patient's body and the adversary of his soul. His efforts to strengthen the one would hasten the corruption of the other, and he would welcome the patient's laughter while lamenting the ruin of his character. A disturbing thought, no doubt. Nevertheless, it is a fact that those theologies that most vehemently attended to the ultimate fate of the soul showed the least solicitude for the concerns of the body, and neglected, if not altogether suppressed, the place assigned to laughter in their doctrines. The coarse pagan gods laughed noisily and at every turn. In this we recognize that they were men, and therefore imperfect: men with magnified powers, thus capable of magnified errors. But in the most spiritual religions the deity attains perfection at the expense of the capacity to laugh. It has been remarked of Christ that he was never known to laugh: He could be sad, or melancholy, or even angry—as when, whip in hand, he chased the merchants from the temple—and he may even be thought of as smiling. But however placid or amiable, his divine demeanor was never convulsed by that mysterious bodily seizure that comforts us in our miseries by blowing away our pains. I mean the hearty, uninhibited, side-splitting laughter. For it would seem that to intellectual perfection, or supreme wisdom, no cause is left for laughter. Our witticisms become transparent wordplay; our comedies, perspicuous absurdities; and our frailties and errors, nothing but the object of commiseration.

It may be that the comic is best left unexplained. Perhaps the most serious mistake is committed by those who would *think* the ludicrous instead of laughing at it. But this in itself is a remarkable fact, and worthy of the most detailed analysis: that there are temperaments fixed in laughless contemplation, and others to which high susceptibility to laughter is connatural. Voltaire noted that the most mirthless of men are always found among those who seek to explain the causes of joy. The ancient Greeks had a word, *agelasti,* to name those who never laughed. It is not that their minds are filled with serious researches and austere thoughts. For the passage from seriousness to laughter is so easy, that it has been contended that the more a man is capable of seriousness, the more he can laugh. Something more basic, more fundamental, lies behind the ability or inability to laugh. There are some who remain convinced that things are as they think them, and that they think them such as they are. Others—blessed be they!—have an eye for the incongruity; at a glance they can spot the discrepancies between thoughts and reality. It is these ones that cannot be made to take the world seriously, and are always ready to laugh.

I will not gainsay the benefits that laughter bestows on the body. No physician who has seen disease put to rout by a mirthful disposition could doubt the awesome power of laughter. But I place little credence in the virtue of jokes dispensed every four hours to all patients. The Norman Cousins experience (which I regard both as a marvelous episode of individual courage and a biologic phenomenon deserving of the fullest investigation) does not affirm, to my mind, the value of humor as medicine. Cousins did not *simply* get better because he laughed, but laughed because he belonged to that courageous segment of mankind that seeks self-affirmation, often in laughter, against all odds. The positive, enthusiastic, vital, laughter-prone faction composed of those who naturally believe that life and the good ultimately shall prevail over death, darkness, and evil. He got well because he was what one may call an optimist; and it was this, his orientation in life, that made him cling to laughter, the badge and banner of the optimist faction. In my opinion (all this is nothing more than opinion), research into the determinants of the innate optimistic disposition would be more fruitful than any amount of investigation into the physiological benefits of laughter. For the optimist condition predates laughter, and may be congenital. Recall that in the dictionary that the Devil dictated to Ambrose Bierce, optimism is described as an inborn affliction curable only by death. And since the Devil works at cross purposes with our designs, he added with a malignant whisper uttered in his croaklike voice that optimism is "also hereditary but, happily, not known to be contagious."

I have very few personal recollections of this kind of recalcitrant optimism. But I know that, when present, it will laugh, and tease, and joke in the very jaws of death. I remember a young Irish immigrant, dying with advanced cancer of rare type, telling me on the day of his death that he only regretted that probably there would be no television sets "where he was going," for he wished to watch a soccer game scheduled for the morrow. Wittier sayings have come from the mouth of the dying, according to trustworthy chroniclers. A humorist who had been a fearsome duellist was on his deathbed in a state of semi-skeletic emaciation after a long illness. Asked by his physician how he felt, he replied: "So weak, that a fly could send me its [duelling] second." Salvator Rosa (1615–1673), Italian painter, musician, poet, and satirist, was admonished by the priest who gave him the last rites to marry his common-law wife, by whom he had fathered children but whom Rosa nonetheless suspected of infidelity. The solemnity of the moment was broken when the dying man said: "Very well. Since you assure me that today one must grow horns to be admitted in heaven, I consent to this marriage."

Would that we were granted that spark, to the very end! To

live with gusto and to die with verve. And to manifest, in the last hour, that neither sickness nor death could take away our capacity to laugh. We may never understand the nature of the comic. We may not have the wit that made a dying humorist say to grieving relatives around him: "You will never cry as much as I made you laugh!" But we can always maintain at least a smile, and that tenor of mind that made Jaquelin des Yveteaux, mediocre poet of the sixteenth century, ask that a lively dance piece be played by musicians in his death chamber.

You see, there are many ways to pass on *allegro*.

ON ANGER, IN IMITATION OF SENECA

Consider the angry man: his face flushed or pale; gait unsteady; speech stuttered; jaws locked and eyes glazed. With tense or tremulous body he staggers, moves erratically, charges against all objects, unafraid of damage to his own frame. Wrath, most conspicuous of the mind's distempers, is also mind's most inimical bent. Which is why the ancient sages laid a double charge at its door, saying that it does offense both to intellect and to esthetics; to the one, because it is impervious to good counsel; to the other, because it always shows up in the face, and is always ugly.

It is a sort of hatred, or aversion against those who have tried to injure us, or to thwart our projects. It is a movement against those who have wronged us, or wished to hurt us. And this is why the ancients could descry a certain sense of retributive justice in this passion, saying that it was the desire to repay evil with evil. Descartes distinguishes it from indignation, which is experienced toward detrimental acts committed against others, and comes mixed with envy, or pity. One becomes indignant at the good of the undeserving, or at the ills of the just; envy thrives in the former case, pity in the latter. Descartes is thus moved to say that "the mockeries of Democritus and the tears of Heraclitus may spring from the same cause." The Cartesian system recognizes, above all, the ease with which anger forms alloys. Admixed with love and kindness, anger becomes vivid, prompt, outward, and easily appeased. But when it combines with sadness, ire is hidden, and we fail to detect the wrathful man, except for pallor in the face; yet, its strength is much enhanced by this combination, and the desire to achieve revenge is heightened.

The Stoics were of a completely different opinion. They could not conceive wrath if not in pure form. Sincere worshippers of reason, they could not imagine the noblest of our functions side by side with a troubling passion. If reason were admixed with anger, they said, it would be weakened by this debasing alliance, and so bastardized it would no longer be capable of containing the impulses it is meant to check. Their tone is derogatory of anger, but never condescending; for no one can deny that this is a passion indomitable, rebellious, and often overpowering. However, they adamantly reject the idea that anger be tolerated in modified form. For there are some who claim that anger may be of practical value; that wrath contains an active principle that stimulates and spurs; and that tempered, but not altogether suppressed, it would suit soldiers in war, or those who must face intimidating dangers. There are some who say that anger may be put at the service of courage, like a dog to the hunter. But anger is not obliging, and will not be measured out in doses. It is either stronger or weaker than reason. If stronger, reason is feeble to keep it abeyant; if weaker, reason alone should suffice for our ends, spurning the assistance of an agent sickly and frail.

It may happen that when a wrathful man is powerful, or his passion extreme, anger assumes an awesome appearance. Do not be deceived: it is never grand. It is all hot air and shameful weakness, even at its most impressive. It is as far from being grand as servility is distant from politeness, rashness from courage, or insolence from familiarity. If you think that anger is majestic, you probably think that luxury and vanity are great, since they are always putting on flashy clothes, traveling in expensive cars, and dwelling amidst superfluous ostentation; or that loan sharks are praiseworthy because they amass great fortunes, own huge tracts of land, and build skyscrapers. You might as well conclude that lasciviousness is a great thing, since many endanger their lives on its account, and risk their social position; since it enslaves men and women, and often ruins the former and prostitutes the latter. It matters not how high-sounding the acquirements of vice may be: its boundaries are set, and are narrow. Pornographers may own multinational corporations. Ruthless men and women may build empires. Profiteers may thrive on the suffering of others, amassing enormous fortunes. But it does not matter that vice trumpets its victories all over the face of the earth, and strikes dreadful reverence in the hearts of millions. It is still base, and petty, and contemptible.[9]

ON DESIRE

In the entire world there is no animal whose appetite for all things exceeds that of man, nor yet is there any that needs so few. To this paradox the sages traced no few of the miseries that afflict us. Seldom do we travel through life unencumbered by a heavy baggage of desires: when young, of pleasures; when middle aged, of honors; and when old, of restitution of lost powers. Each of us is impelled by a kind of thirst to secure what our judgment values as the highest good at every moment. But this great number of desires is not surprising, since only that which is lacking is desired. And our natures are so limited and imperfect, that scarcely a moment goes by without a new desire manifesting itself, and urging us, implacably, to give it satisfaction.

Spinoza placed desire as the cornerstone of all passions, for the reason that somehow there must be an appetite for injuring others in hatred, or for seeking their good in love, or for avoiding them in fear. He makes no distinction between appetite and desire, a synonymy that some deem less than perfect. In his *Ethics,* he notes that there is nothing that men are less able to do than to control the emergence of their appetites (Part III, proposition 2). Accordingly, ethics must place desire at the very core of our being. In the Spinozian definition, "desire is the essence itself of man in so far as it is conceived as determined to any action by one of his affections" (prop. 59). Thus, fear is the desire of avoiding ills, benevolence the desire to favor those whom we pity, avarice the immoderate desire of riches, and so on. And many have said, without fear of making distorted exaggerations, that all human actions spring from desires which are anterior to any calculation of pleasure and pain. Bertrand Russell must be counted among believers in the prepotency of desire, since he reduced the whole field of ethics to a series of volitional statements. He thought that the concept of good and evil would best be removed from logic, for it cannot be dealt with in the same way as a logical proposition. Men would save themselves countless troubles, he said, if they read ethical statements as statements of desires of the propounder. Thus, when someone says, "it is good to be honest and wrong to cheat," the sensible listener should not take this statement as he would a statement that can be proved by logical argument. Rather, he ought to know that all the expositor is trying to do is to manifest this desire: "Would that all were honest and that no one would cheat!"

In the beginning there was desire.

Amidst all this flattery of desire and admission of its importance, one voice dissents. Alain,[10] who feared nothing and desired so little, felt no respect for desire, and saw no place for "this little personage" among the passions. For instance, the true passion for gambling he saw as made entirely of fear, and possibly as an exercise to overcome it. But, as to desire, it is nowhere to be seen. "Whosoever desires to win, also desires not to lose; and it would be ridiculous to see desire by the gambling table. Win or lose: it is of no consequence. Do not confuse the need to play the game with the desire to win." And love? Does not the lover desire his beloved? Here, too, a subtle difference is introduced. The true lover pays no attention to the means and the beginnings: he is projected, impelled forwards by a kind of wave, toward the unforeseeable. But desire is anticipation and planning: it calculates and prearranges what is to be said in a future conversation. "Such a road leads to despising," says Alain, whereas the royal road of love leads to will the love-object happy, free, and powerful. "I say to will, not to desire: there is an immense difference between the expectation of a perfection, and the action that wantonly grabs it to emplace it."

Curious, indeed, Alain's subtle distinction between willing, needing, and desiring. One may ask, where would the field of ethics be if Alain had been less of a poet and more of a philosopher?

ON WEEPING

Grief is the opposite of joy, as tears are the opposite of laughter. A greater commotion is triggered in the face by the agency of grief than by mirth. The corners of the mouth are drawn down, and the eyebrows become oblique because of the lifting and puckering of their inner ends. The forehead develops central vertical and transverse furrows resembling a triangle.

In happiness, it is chiefly the zygomatic muscles that contract. But in the creation of the sad face many muscles must be contracted: the elevators, orbicularis oculi, orbicularis oris, corrugator, frontalis, pyramidal, and many more. Thus popular wisdom maintains, not without foundation, that a happy face looks young because it is easily maintained, whereas frequent crying is harsh toil that desolates the face and promotes premature wrinkles.

Nevertheless grief is the first, then the only, and, for some time, the most frequently manifested emotion. With the admirable tenacity of researchers, the frequency of weeping in early life has been counted.[11] Crying episodes occur approximately four thousand times during the first two years of life. Toward this phenomenon, however, society is highly inconsistent. Our arrival into the world is marked by crying, by uttering as loud a wail as could be expected of someone who has lived minutes, or seconds. This cry evokes generalized rejoicing. But as soon as we become teachable it is impressed upon us that crying is unseemly. Of weeping, an English ophthalmologist had this to say: "The conventions of Anglo-Saxon civilization have latterly imposed an excessive husbandry on so natural a physiological release."[12] The most obedient among us learn the lesson. And then, when ready to exit from life, their composed departure takes place amidst universal weeping.

What does all this muscular activity mean, this "discomposing" of the face that composes a crying face? Darwinians explain that some animals' snarl is a threatening gesture, by which they display their fangs and so intimidate potential foes. But do we mean to threaten when we smile, or grin and bare our teeth? And what possible advantage could we have derived in millennia of evolutionary adaptation by displaying the tempestuous grimacing of grief? A brave theorist of emotional expression, Israel Waynbaum, supplied an original explanation. Muscles of the face are brought into action, he stated, to compress blood vessels of the head and thus to regulate blood flow to the brain. Arteries to the brain and to the face arise from a common source, the common carotid artery. This vessel, in turn, divides into two main branches, one to be distributed in the face, and the other in the brain. The circulatory blood flow to the brain must be kept constant, or nearly so, lest sudden drops plunge us into unconsciousness, or abrupt rises into apoplexy. The face, in contrast, allows for brusque and important variations: we blush and we pale with the greatest of ease. To Waynbaum, the many muscles of the face exist for a purpose—namely, for compressing, like tourniquets, the vessels of the head against the facial skeleton. By this means, the blood may be diverted toward the face or toward the brain, depending on the needs imposed by the emotional state.

In Waynbaum's hypothesis the affective tone of the individual is maintained by a system of dikes and sluice doors monitored by the muscles of expression. During the act of smiling, the muscles that pull the lips act also as ligatures on the branches of the facial arteries. This causes greater influx of blood to the brain, which may explain the subjective feeling of elation. Strenuous laughter turns the face red, or as purple as a beet, on account of the impedance to venous outflow produced by cervical skin muscles compressing the jugular veins. The result is that more blood is retained in the brain, thus increasing the affective tone. The opposite would be observed during sadness, or depression. Energy demands are lowered, and circulatory adjustment diverting blood away from the brain would reduce blood flow, producing a negative affective tone, and perhaps also some degree of anesthesia. And tears? At the end of a bout of loud laughter, they are the product of secretion of glands engorged with blood, and thus a means of alleviating cerebral congestion. If prompted by sadness, the activity of the lacrimal glands is still mediated by the action of the muscles of facial expression compressing the blood vessels.

This theory, which at first impresses us as a coarse mechanistic view by an imaginative physiologist of the last century, has been recently vindicated. In a recent issue of the prestigious journal *Science,* Professor Zajonc, of the University of Michigan, "reclaimed" Waynbaum's theory for the attention of contemporary researchers.[13] Allowance made for certain unwarranted assumptions and factual errors (inevitable, given the state of development of science at the time of its framing), this theory, we are told, adequately accounts for observable facts of emotional expression, and does so more satisfactorily than either Darwinian concepts or psychological explanations. For instance, actors instructed to reproduce the facial expressions associated with, say, fear or disgust, manifest involuntary bodily changes that are regularly associated with such emotions. Over these concomitants, like pulse rate or blood pressure, we are ordinarily powerless. Thus, Professor Zajonc sees here a just occasion to reexamine Waynbaum's concepts. In artificially creating the face of fear, or disgust, the actors' facial muscles might be compressing blood vessels and readjusting blood flow to the brain. The net result could be the observed involuntary effects upon the autonomic nervous system.

A corollary of this would be that training individuals prone to depression to control their facial musculature may have the beneficial effect of predisposing them to more positive affective states. Zajonc points out that Yoga and various forms of meditation attempt to attain precisely this result. It is perhaps unnecessary to refer to Eastern meditation techniques; popular wisdom among us enjoins us to "put on a happy face" in adversity, clearly recognizing the effect on mood of facial expression. The tradition is an old one. Plutarch, in his *Consolation to His Wife* upon the death of their daughter Timoxena, criticizes mourners who neglect the care of their bodies, showing aversion to ointment, the bath, and other usages proper to daily life. His advice is to do precisely the opposite, for suffering loses its cutting angles "when dissipated in the calm of the body, as waves are dispersed in fair weather."[14] Conversely, if the body is allowed to grow squalid and unkempt, it will send up to the soul "only pains, like acrid and noisome exhalations"; and then the soul becomes so firmly gripped by suffering, that easy recovery is no longer possible even when desired. Here we have described, in the first century of our era, what today's technological partiality would no doubt call "a feedback mechanism."

Whatever may be the salutary physiological effects of laughter, or weeping, it remains unsolved why some are unusually prone, and others resistant, to these outbursts. Yet more intriguing, but equally unexplained, is the fact that some laugh when others weep, and some weep at what makes others laugh. Pliny reported that Phocion was never known to weep, or to laugh (*Nat. Hist.* 7:19). The Greek philosopher Heraclitus wept at everything that occurred. Democritus of Abdera, on the contrary, laughed ceaselessly at the spectacle of the world. Their contemporaries pitied the former and were angered at the latter, whom they considered mad. Hippocrates was consulted to diagnose the ailment of the laughing man, but declared, after taking the clinical history, that Democritus was the very picture of health. Otherwise stated, the case may be made in earnest that the world is eminently funny. There were no requests for medical consultation on behalf of the weeping philosopher. From which we may gather that the free citizens of classical Greece, like our contemporaries, were readier to tolerate those who were crushed by the system, than those perceptive enough to laugh at its follies. I have no doubt that today we would declare the one manic, and the other depressive. We have created a world separated from universal nuclear destruction by a hair's breadth, marred by social injustices of every description, and racked with the appalling consequences of our own improvidence. This world we are asked to observe, on pain of societal punishment, with perfect impassiveness and untroubled equanimity. For the reactions of men who, like Democritus and Heraclitus, are all too perceptive and uninhibited, we have a label: "inappropriate emotional response."

Considering the nature of contemporary societies, and of our emotional makeup, it seems to me that the temperament best suited to make life tolerable would be a hybrid one. It ought to be made of a combination of personages that I find quoted by Laurent Joubert in his *Treatise on Laughter:*[15] Phocion, who never wept; Nerva, who never played; Marcus Crassus, who never laughed; Antonia, wife of Drusus, who never spat; Pomponius, consular poet, who never burped. Comments Joubert: "all of which things nevertheless seem proper to man."

Three Theorists
of Emotion

RENÉ DESCARTES

To the modern biologist, the name of René Descartes may seem out of place in the company of explorers of the mechanism of emotions. But it was precisely as a physician, or physiologist, that he wrote that wonderful little volume, so often quoted, yet so little read, to which he gave the expressive title of *Treatise on the Passions of the Soul.* He wrote the book, as he said in his correspondence with Princess Elizabeth, daughter of the Elector Palatine, not from the point of view of the philosopher, or scientist, but from the medical point of view. It is not Descartes the moralist who speaks; it is Descartes the physician.[1]

Another source of impatience for the modern reader lies with some of Descartes's major premises. One is his reasoning that leads to the famous paradox of living beings as nothing but mechanical contrivances. But one must understand the notions that the philosopher had to sort out in his difficult meditation. How could the soul, the mind, be said to be dependent on the body? Mind is what "comprehends" all things, all bodies—their differences, their extent, and their number. Could such an entity, surpassing the immensity of all things, be said to be confined by the narrow limits of a body, and, in a sense, subservient to the needs of the body? True to his faith in consistency and logic, Descartes could never admit such incongruence. Rather, his courageous answer was this, that the soul has its own physiology, and the activities of the body are pure mechanical gadgetry. Breathing, walking, eating, and generally "all activities which we share in common with unthinking beasts" are produced exclusively as a result of the peculiar conformation of our bodily parts, and the excitation that certain stimulatory substances exert upon them. He chose to name these substances "animal spirits" *(esprits animaux)*. Replace the name with current scientific terms: acetylcholine, endorphin, serotonin, DOPA, whatever you like, and much of Cartesian thought could pass for a contemporary production. But, as to his fundamental view of bodily workings, his position was taken: all that happens in our body is comparable to the activities of a clock that has been wound (This terminology also needs updating; today we would say "like a computer that has been programmed"). Its motions derive solely from the strength of the winding mechanism and the arrangement of its springs and wheels—nothing more. All is accomplished by the body, without the assistance of the soul.

As to animals, who have no soul, they are automata. Only men have souls, he said, and only thoughts constitute the soul's activity. This is the Cartesian statement that animal lovers will not forgive. For they deem it a most uncharitable notion to deny that animals exhibit sentiments of admiration, love, pity, or jealousy. Is it not love that moves a dog to wag its tail and jump excitedly at the approach of its master? Go tell a pet owner that his parrot does not recognize him, or that the purring of his cat is not a grateful acknowledgment of kindness received! But Descartes is inflexible. They are robots. And his supporters—for this French gentleman still has them, and of the highest merit —have summoned one argument that even today strikes me as overwhelming. If you truly believe that animals have a soul, what possible justification can you give to the centuries-old holocaust, the continuing, daily, bloody sacrifice of millions and millions of animals, for the sake of man's welfare, appetite, pride, or vanity?

In order to examine Descartes's ideas on emotion, let us now advance what is perhaps emotion's most quoted scenario. An enraged dog, barking furiously, bristling and foaming at the mouth, appears down the street and charges at us. Our pupils dilate, our hair stands on end, our hearts beat faster, and we run for dear life. Or a rival insults us with abrading words. We attempt to retort, but the rascal is too quick-witted for us. We are left speechless and humiliated. Then, our veins dilate, our vision blurs, and our muscles tense. Angry and "beside ourselves," we strike. In each case a mental perception has triggered an amazing array of involuntary bodily activities. Evidently, a mental process is all that is required. Our foe need not be present. A mere recollection of his past impertinence would suffice to make us angry. The raging dog may be wholly imaginary, a hallucination; we would be no less frightened. And the question that arises is, how is it possible for these bodily discharges to become real? We know they normally exist as potentiality in our psychic life. But we wish to know how it comes about that our lives, that we fancy normally calm and subdued, should be periodically shaken by these inner crises, these tremors.

The Cartesian system, with all its outmoded notions of physiology, contains the basic elements of insight upon which others have built their theories. For Descartes, the perception of a "strange and frightful animal" approaching us is transmitted to the pineal gland, and this "disposes the brain in such a way that the 'spirits' reflected from the image thus formed on the gland proceed to take their places partly in the nerves which serve to turn the back and dispose the legs for flight, and partly in those which so increase or diminish the orifices of the heart . . . [that it] sends to the brain the 'spirits' which are adapted for the maintenance and strengthening of the passion of fear" (Art. 36). Moreover, the persistent influx of "spirits" to the pineal causes the "soul to be sensible to this passion."

Fright, therefore, is an awareness of the changes in the body tending to cause us to flee. Insofar as it is an awareness, emotion is knowledge. The emotion may have been triggered by a perception (and then, of course, by memory, since it is requisite to identify a frightful object as damaging, by comparison with previously experienced hurtful objects), but perception is not emotion. The emotion does not arise until the commotions of the body become registered as a *feeling*. The Cartesian definition of emotion may thus be put in these words: Emotion is the reflective awareness, by the soul, of the mechanical commotions going on in the body. It is an awareness and a feeling.

It is easy to forgive him for his rudimentary notions of physiology; there was, after all, no better science in his day. And there is a serene beauty in his reasoning that the soul must exert its functions most particularly in that little gland (pineal) embedded in the substance of the brain, as if "suspended" at the crossroads of its inner cavities (Art. 31). Why should our contemporaries deride this conclusion? If today's scientists take for granted that the whole emotional domain resides in neurophysiology, it was not so in Descartes's time, when the heart was assumed to be the principal seat of emotion. To have uprooted this received opinion was no mean achievement, all the more admirable when one considers that he did it with no other tools than his splendid, lucid reasoning (Art. 33). So what, if he chooses to make the pineal gland the seat of the soul (Art. 32)? Modern reference to this is usually sarcastic, as if it had been a lunatic's raving. But then, few read today the noble paragraphs, the superb effort that explains: "All the parts of our brain are double, as are the eyes, the hands, the ears and the organs of our senses; and, inasmuch as we have a single thought of a single thing at any one time, there must be a place where the two images that come through the eyes, or the two impressions that come through duplicated organs of sense, could gather [before exciting the soul] . . . but there is no place in the organism where they could be so joined, if it is not this little gland." The test of ideas is truthfulness or falsity, but scoffing has no part in the evaluation. And if it is to be doled out at all, it clearly should go to efforts less noble and splendid than those of René Descartes.

Nevertheless, the Cartesian system of the emotions left itself open to criticism in proposing that the soul was a passive agent (hence the term "passion" for emotion) in the turmoil of the body. He would have us believe that the feeling of this excitation "disposes" the will to action: to flee from the enraged dog, or to attack the offending rival. But it has been validly countered that a feeling, in fact, disposes to nothing. Descartes does not tell us how a certain "awareness of the bodily commotions going on" links itself with desire and behavior. Nor does he explain, other than by passing reference to "different internal temperaments," why it is that the same stimulus disposes some to fight, others to flight.

WILLIAM JAMES

James[2] is very much a Cartesian. He begins by telling us that no emotion is possible without the body's involuntary functions —that winding mechanism in the clock. Take these away, and human life freezes into a kind of icicle that no one, apart from Kant and the ancient Stoics, ever considered possible, or desirable. For then each of the mental perceptions that arouse the emotions would become mere acts of intellectual cognition. Let the raging dog charge at us. We would simply become aware that a threatening beast is coming our way and that, in consequence, it would be prudent to flee. Let the rival offend us. We would become aware of the offense, and allow that some kind of retaliatory action is called for, to even the scores. But there would be no quickened pulse, no flushing of the face, no rapid breathing, no horripilation, no cold sweat. In one word, no emotion. In place of emotion we would have judgment, calculation, cognition: anything but emotion.

This point is insistently reiterated: The organic discharge *is* the emotion. William James hammers it down, knowing full well that acceptance of this premise is essential for all that follows. When one reads the first half of his famous monographic article, "The Emotions," one gets the impression that the author is getting ready to make a paradoxical statement, knowingly. He sounds like one who is about to introduce a frumpish guest to a fastidious group of snobs—the readers—and justifies his action in advance. He clears the ground. Let the reader abstract from his consciousness, he says, all feelings of bodily symptoms connected with fright, and then tell us, in all honesty, whether there is anything left that might constitute an emotion. Take away the sweaty palms, the "goose flesh," and so on, and then tell us what "mind stuff" is left that could be called emotion.

Having made his point abundantly clear, James is ready for the controversial statement: "Common sense says, we lose our fortune, are sorry and weep; we meet a bear, are frightened and run; we are insulted by a rival, are angry and strike ... [but] one mental state is not immediately induced by the other, ... the bodily manifestations must first be interposed between, and the more rational statement is that we feel sorry because we cry, angry because we strike, afraid because we tremble, and not that we cry, strike or tremble, because we are sorry, angry or fearful, as the case may be."

Here is the paradox. James and his followers blatantly disregard what we call "common sense." And this is always a risky and ungrateful task. They are intent in showing that the bodily reactions are triggered *before* the intellectual cognition that common sense stubbornly keeps placing at their start. And you cannot catch them off guard, their hands empty of supporting examples. Thus, James reminds us that a child manifests the full range of the emotion of fright even *before* he can discern the actual threat in the object that frightens it; that a dimly perceived object startles us; that the shadow of a man in a solitary place affrights us *before* we can find reasons for our alarm. And the sight of blood, as is well known, is capable of triggering severe involuntary reactions, including fainting spells, even in persons fully aware that the bleeding is insignificant and poses no threat. For James, the bodily changes follow directly the perception of the exciting fact by a kind of natural ("preorganized," he says; "preprogrammed," again we might say) predisposition. And when these bodily changes are felt, the emotion is experienced.

So we can see that James, whether he knew it or not, is Cartesian to the core. Emotions to him are just awareness of bodily sensations. In other words, *feelings* of physiological phenomena that are in turn triggered by perceptions. With one difference, however. That whereas Descartes took away the emotions from the body and made them a part of the physiology of the soul, James took the emotion away from the soul and placed it squarely within the purview of the body's physiology. James was the first to contend that, since the bodily discharge *is* the emotion, the study of the emotions should be made a branch of physiology. The corollary is self-evident: differences between emotions are based on differences between physiological reactions. If we only knew with scientific precision the quantitative and qualitative differences that exist in the physiological reactions of a happy and a saddened man, we would fully understand happiness and sadness. And if we could find out the changes in cardiac activity, glandular secretion, nervous transmission, etc., in other emotional states, we would have the key to love, hate, anger, fright, and the whole retinue of "passions."

The flaws in the theory are now well known. The physiologic changes present in an angered man are not radically different from those of an ecstatically happy one: in both, breathing is rapid, resistance to fatigue is enhanced, metabolic pace accelerates, blood pressure rises, and so on. The more we know about this, the more the conclusion is strengthened that Cannon[3] was correct when he interpreted his experimental work as indicating that the reactions of the body overlap in different emotions. Or, as a more recent investigator put it, "the same visceral changes occur in very different emotional states, and in non-emotional states."[4] Thus, the bodily reactions are the same, but the projection of these reactions to our consciousness registers as radically different. Could it be that the differences are of a quantitative kind? Even if this were the case, the differences in experienced emotion are so vast, that we would be forced to look for a more satisfactory explanation. Few researchers would summon the courage to tell a betrayed, angry lover that, because his bodily reactions are only quantitatively different and of higher magnitude than those of his successful rival, science considers him to be "extra-happy."

Whatever his detractors might say, there is no little beauty, and all the appeal of paradoxes, in James's theory. For it seems to turn our bodies into string instruments that the environment dexterously plays on. I see the perfect mutual adequacy of performer and instrument. For the stimuli that excite the emotions are not directed at random. James does not expressly deny emotions to the higher animals. Thus, living beings appear as instruments uniquely adapted to the hands of nature-as-virtuoso. The proximity of a precipice will pluck reverberating notes of vertigo in man, but not in bird or in mountain goat. The sight of an egg nest will have no emotional content for us, but will sound we know not what nurturing-love resonance in eagle, lark, or sparrow. And the note will be amplified, as by a resonance box, in the living organism. The complexity of the emotional response will accrue of itself thanks to the natural properties of the body.

This idea is not new in James. Diderot spoke of our nerves as vibrating strings that are, in addition, sensitive. And if vibrating strings of an instrument, inert and separate, communicate their vibrations to adjacent strings, "how can this fail to take place between parts that are living and linked to each other, sensitive and continuous?" The theory, therefore, is a "peripheralist" one. It views emotions as the result of the excitation of our sense organs, amplified by the body. Our sense organs are tended to the outer world, like tense strings. And like strings in a musical instrument, they are plucked by the ever-changing phenomena of the environment around us, much as if by the nimble fingers of a soloist.

JEAN PAUL SARTRE

The *coup de grâce* was delivered to the "peripheralist" theory not by a psychologist, as expected, but by a philosopher. It was Sartre[5] who first noted that, if emotions were preset bodily reactions to perceived stimuli (presumably fixed by millennia of evolution, and thus having a survival value), it would be very difficult to explain the apparently counterproductive effect of some emotional states. Upon seeing the ferocious dog charging at me, it seems appropriate that I should react with the emotions that best prepare me for fight or flight: either the tonus for combat, or the mental climate for escape. Instead, it may happen that I freeze in terror; I am not fit for one or the other. Worse than that. My legs, which should have stood firm to repel the attack or kept nimble to take me away from danger, seem to melt, wobble, and turn weak. And my circulatory system, which should have assisted me in my defense, fails me as well. Some defense! A fainting spell seems, at this juncture, the least appropriate behavior. Surely, evolutionary striving did not imprint on me *this* reaction to help me through the biologic struggle.

But the Sartrian explanation sees here a purposeful design. Since I had tried to evade the danger, but had no way to succeed, I opted to deny the existence of danger. I have *willed* the disappearance of the threat. And I have done this by resorting to magic. "Let there be no more ferocious dog," I have pronounced, becoming suddenly a demiurge, or a magician. And the danger ceased to be. And this does not mean that it has simply ceased to exist for me. I am convinced that I have achieved a fundamental transmutation of the world of reality. Absurd? You bet: absurd under the normal sequences of logic. But perfectly possible "by magic"—that is, outside of the world of normal deterministic logical sequences. Berkeley would have loved Sartre's theory. For if it is true, as Berkeley affirmed, that material things exist only as objects of thought—that is, as contents of some consciousness—then there can be no more effective way of erasing an undesirable reality than by annihilating consciousness.

I remember a professor of mine, a choleric individual who would bully his assistants, tear up documents in their presence, and hurl pieces of equipment against the wall, leaving his contrite students to pick up the debris when he had quit the room, after slamming the door. In the normal, rational world, his behavior could not have been more absurd. But in the world of magic that Sartre would have us assume, his acts were perfectly consistent. Having failed to achieve his ends, having failed to circumvent each obstacle that stood in his way, what else was left but to charge furiously, blindly, to shatter in pieces the hindrances that still stood? I only saw him falter and lose face once. This was when, directing his fulminations to a young woman, she reacted with convulsive sobs and loud cries. It seemed to us that an irascible man had been confounded by an emotionally unstable girl. But the Sartrian explanation would have been less simple. The girl could be seen as *willing* the magic transformation of a ruthless tyrant, deaf to appeals, into a sympathetic listener, or at least a neutral agent. What others had failed to accomplish by conventional ways, she did by magic. "I will not be bullied. You will cease to be the irate aggressor that you are," she seemed to be saying. And this statement was not a verbal one, for she was in no condition to hold a verbal dialogue. She used all her body—convulsing with emotion—to unhinge the rigid behavior of the professor. No one had ever succeeded before in accomplishing that task. But this in no way means that she was "faking," or playing a comedy. Far from that. Her sobs, her tears, her pallor, her trembling fully attested to what Sartre called "the body's belief in its magical conduct." For Sartre also noted that "emotion is a matter of belief . . . and to believe in magic one has to be moved."

If there is a theory of emotion with what one might call "esthetic" appeal, it is certainly this one. It has all the elegance of a probing into the unconscious, and all the mystery of an invocation of the world of magic and the occult. It is almost a pedestrian anticlimax to point out that there are objections to its postulates.

Above all, it may have been a mistake for Sartre to use the example of swooning in the face of overwhelming danger. For in so doing, he committed himself to presenting a view of emotions as misguided, aberrant, or plain misfiring mental processes. This has been pointed out in a brilliant study of emotions by the philosopher William Lyons.[6] Sartre's view, notes Lyons, is "[that] the emotional behavior results, not from an accurate view of some event in the world and an assessment of what is to be done about it, but from a failure to cope with some event in the world, which failure generates an illusory view of the event." But it is by no means established that emotional behavior is always that chaotic, or disorganized, or misguided sort of activity. True enough, I may fall prey to a fainting attack when I see the dog at my heels. But this is not the necessary consequence of that situation. Nor can I summon at will the singular means of escape. And while it is true that the emotional response makes us act *as if* we searched for a magical solution, it is also true that oftentimes we react appropriately to lucidly perceived circumstances. It is a fact proved by experience that when spurred by fright we run faster, and when goaded by wrath we strike harder. And one may reasonably propose that beneficial outcomes, issuing (as they most commonly do) from a swift and accurate assessment of real circumstances, are likelier consequences of stress than "a fall into the world of magic."

AN EPILOGUE (OF SORTS)

I have chosen to present three theories on emotion. I hope not to be blamed if I confess that the choice was based on esthetics over testable veracity. The virtue of the theories is, to my mind, beauty. They please on account of their comprehensiveness and, not surprisingly, they are owed to philosophers. (I do not hesitate in including William James in this category, nor do I think he would have disclaimed it.) Psychologists, and scientists generally, appear to be too busy with partial aspects that constantly and uncontrollably spring up, like mushrooms, in their fertile fields of specialization. The trite comparison is to see these fields as leading upwards. But it is hard to avoid the feeling that they must be sloping downwards, in steep declivity, seeing that no one seems to have the chance to pause for a moment in the fatal race of discoveries, to determine how they all connect in a rounded account of the human being. Nor do I apologize to philosophers for my amateurish incursion onto their turf. They know very well that theirs is not an exclusive property, but one whose value rises in proportion as it is kept open for the public. The amateur will bungle, and lose his way, and look rather sorry when he is done treading the unfamiliar paths. But the philosopher is a benevolent landowner. He smiles at the clumsiness of the visitor and then smiles again, less condescendingly, when the visitor leaves the toll on which the keeper of the grounds depends for his livelihood, a small, shiny coin: a fresh look, an original perception, "for what it's worth."

As a physician, I never felt very comfortable in the company of the three illustrious theorists. Descartes was polite and ceremonious, and I was charmed by his courtly manner and polished language. But he spoke to me from an era when the circulation of the blood was just being discovered, and held, I thought, rather exotic views on physiology. James was almost poetical in some parts of his exposition, but I simply could not swallow his belief that the bodily alterations and the emotion are the same thing. For I know that the injection of certain drugs (and today we have innumerable pharmacologic agents) can reproduce virtually all the concomitants of emotion without the subject manifesting that he feels saddened, or joyful, or in love. At most, as with hallucinogens, he might manifest a quasi-pathologic euphoria, or depression, that stands in relation to the emotions of joy and sadness as a caricature to a portrait. And then, it seems that the body has but a limited supply of overlapping symptoms to express an unlimited range of emotions. Whatever the subtlety of an emotion, it seems always to come out via the "final common pathway" of goose bumps, palpitations, high blood pressure, pupillary changes, and *few* other symptoms. Finally, with Mr. Sartre I was like a timid man with a phobia for heights, tied to an intellectual roller coaster. I could hardly follow the vigorous mind in those stupendous caroms and revolutions. If, sometimes, I was swept up by the divine afflatus, I felt something akin to vertigo or the bends. But when the ride was over, I could not avoid resettling into the prosaic clinical mode. And this unpoetical frame of mind kept telling me that the person who faints under highly stressful circumstances does so because of some sudden derangement in the neurophysiology that controls the waking state—and nothing more. In other words, what occurs is a sudden disruption of the physiologic mechanisms that control consciousness, *without* the need to invoke the world of magic.

I suppose my position is clear. I take leave of philosophers, and claim the province of emotion as the rightful estate of scientists—for now. For the time being, I believe, the claim lies with physiologists, or neurobiologists. In the future, probably, with physicists. Does this mean that philosophers are being evicted from their ancestral homestead? This property, these grounds that they so generously made available to the public, are they going to be confiscated without so much as a token indemnity? Hardly. The "squatters" may think so, but here is where I part company with my fellow clinicians.

Assume, for the sake of the argument, that the scientists' job is complete. Never mind that this will take thousands of years: we are not in a hurry. Assume, then, that every molecular event in the brain is fully and exhaustively known. Every "transmitter," every "receptor," every "mediator," in every nook and cranny of the brain, finally understood. Not merely in sketch, but to the last detail of molecular, atomic, and subatomic particle arrangement. It is not inconceivable that the fluid activities of the mind could also come under the consummate and final scientific scrutiny. For the information derived from millions of simultaneous probes could be continuously monitored, stored, and analyzed by the super-efficient computers of the future. Picture this scenario and then consider the experiment that is about to take place. A man, the experimental subject, lies recumbent, surrounded by the neurosurgeons of the future. I do not know whether they will opt to cut a circular trephine in the man's head, or whether they will have found ways to circumvent the need for this hinged opercular top. But this point is of no relevance to our argument. The fact is, the scientists peek at the brain, and collect the overwhelming mass of scientific data that the man's brain generates. Which data are transmitted via the sophisticated recorders to the computers.

I now ask, would any examination of the billions of data thus gathered suffice to tell us what was the content of the thoughts of the experimental subject? Could we, by analysis of this information, tell what the gist of his emotional feelings was at a particular time? The question is perhaps idle, but I think the answer is no. I grant the possibility that this hypothetical laboratory experiment one day might tell us, in a general way, whether the subject experiences a positive or a negative feeling. But no amount of faith in the powers of science can persuade me that we would know whether he is gripped by jealousy, wafted by joy, corroded by envy, or vibrating, like a well-tempered violin, to the harmonious chords of love. As to the contents of his non-emotional thoughts, I truly doubt that the ultra-sophisticated paraphernalia could distinguish between the man who thinks a theorem, composes a symphony, or regrets that his soup was cold.

And if our sophisticated recorders gave us measurable data, could we measure the intensity of an emotion? In *Either/Or*, Kierkegaard gathers a panel of judges around an empty tomb inscribed "The Unhappiest Man."[7] The right of occupying it is to be awarded to the claimant with the pitiable distinction of being the unhappiest. What follows is a prolix examination of sadness. A disheveled, red-eyed young woman, her face covered with ashes and her garments torn, stands in front of the judges and states her claim. She is the betrayed lover. All her hopes, all her reasons for living, were once placed in love. Yet she was betrayed, and all that sustained her life is taken away from her. Is she the unhappiest? Other claimants appear before the judges. The deliberation starts. Is the saddest he who loves what he lost in the past, but can remember having had it, and thus finds comfort in memory? Or is it the one who loses his love in the present, but can still hope, and therefore finds solace in the future? Or is the greater sadness that which hopes for something while knowing that it can have no reality in the future? Is it not worse to hope for the unrealizable in the future, at the same time that one has forgotten the past? Is the saddest man, then, one who travels through life unaware of its pleasures, but discovers them on his deathbed, and then *does not die?*

Read the magnificent paragraphs in Kierkegaard, and then tell me whether you think that the solution to the problem of The Unhappiest Man is just one of the potential applications of the computer.

The point is, I believe, that after we are done with the inventory of every possible parameter measurable by science, we will still lack the key to our thoughts and emotions. Behind the scientifically detectable activities of the mind, there will still be *something.* What this something may be it would be presumptuous of me to try to guess, but I believe it should be given a name. We cannot talk about it as "nothing," since we admit that it is something. There are some die-hards that speak of it as "the soul," but they are a negligible minority. Those with a taste for obscure terminology are ready to propose "entelechia," or some such. The problem with such words is that they are not sharable, and, if we used them, soon we would not know what we were talking about. I suppose that in the future world that we are imagining enough wisdom would exist for wanton coining of words like "entelechia" to have been officially declared a misdemeanor subject to harsh penalties. Hegelians and phenomenologists might still exist, but only as secret societies shunned by the worthiest members of the community. Thus, we would have to use such expressions as "the illusory projection of our wishes," "a figment of the imagination," "a ghost," or "a shadow." I will settle for a shadow, as pithier and easier to remember.

The conclusion is clear. In the future world, thousands of years hence, there will still be shadows to chase. Let this be reassurance to poets and philosophers. For they exercise the two trades whose main business is shadow-hunting.

Some Expressions
of the Body
(in Four Movements)

ALLEGRO VIVACE

Look at the body. In the functioning of its parts there is a marvelous congruence, a perfect equality that annexes beauty to utility, so that we are at a loss whether first to admire the one or praise the other. "Harmony" was the Greek word invented to denote this admirable coordination. And it is proper that the word be also a musical term, for just as sounds that accord with each other are immediately perceived as delightful, and those discordant as irksome, so the agreement or discrepancy of the motions of an individual body is immediately seized by the mind before there is any need for reflection. Destroy this harmony, and the expression of the body becomes complex, cryptic, pitiable, or laughable.

Consider the principle of suppleness present in the body's every activity. It confers on every motion, on every gesture, the virtue of opportuneness and the grace of nimbleness. In response to every change in the conditions of the environment, our body summons the appropriate, exquisitely monitored reflex. But in the measure that this spontaneity is destroyed, we come to resemble puppets or mechanical contraptions. Bergson saw here the origin of hilarity: "the mechanic superimposed on life." The insistent mannerisms, tics, reiterative gestures, are invariably comic. For this automatism transforms an independent and well-coordinated being into a puppet jerking at the pulls of strings, over which it has no control. The most solemn ceremony loses its imposing aura when its pomp is viewed as automatism. Abstract all symbolism from it, and it will strike you as a ludicrous charade: the magistrates with their gowns, the generals with their uniforms, the affected curtsies, the ceremonial pacing, all will seem eminently comic, like the awkwardly rigid responses of a group of marionettes.

An Italian humorist, Achille Campanile,[1] exploited the comical in the body's automatism. In his novel, *L'Eroe,* this is carried to its last and most absurd consequences. A young man loses an arm and is fitted with an artificial one. But the prosthesis is defective: the mechanism of its joints, activated by a system of springs, tends to be triggered by minor trepidations, and sometimes becomes jammed. On the day that the Fascist regime of Italy is overturned, the young man finds himself on streets coursed by truckloads of excited demonstrators eager to spill the blood of Nazi sympathizers. Ideological passions have reached the boiling point. The slightest wrong movement could spell death. As luck would have it, the prosthetic joint is activated precisely at this moment, and the artificial arm shoots up in a straight, rigid posture indistinguishable from the Roman, or Fascist salute. Our young man escapes death at the hands of an irate mob, but suffers seven years' imprisonment.

The end of his prison term is about to arrive, when new troubles erupt. Armed revolutionists attempting a *coup d'état* forcibly take the prison on the day that the young man faces the parole-board officers and is about to be released. The enraged rebels clamor at the prison doors, when the prosthetic joints' mechanism jams again. It is the Fascist salute! Feverishly, the prison officers work to bend the rigid artificial fingers, afraid to be surprised by the excited mutineers in the company of an unregenerate political outcast. The result of their efforts is depressing: the closed-fist salute now looks like the Communists' salute, and it is known to all that the rebels are ferociously anti-Communist. One desperate suggestion is made: what if the poor wretch is left to exhibit the Fascist salute with one arm, and the Communist salute with the other? But this cancelling-out scheme (by which the result would add up, presumably, to political neutrality) has one danger. The man could be taken for an opportunist, and all would be massacred. Another idea: the hand should be half-open and half-shut, folding some fingers and extending others. Frantic efforts are again exerted to achieve this result. Alas, this will not do. Now the salute looks like a Churchillian V. He will be taken for a warmonger, an Anglophile, a Quisling, a colonialist. All join their efforts to modify the position of the fingers. Mercy! The gesture becomes that of a priest blessing the faithful. He and his companions will be branded pro-clerical, reactionary, bigoted, fanatic, papists. They are as good as dead. New frantic efforts to rework the position of the fingers. In their haste, however, they ruin the hinge mechanism. Now a single finger, the middle one, is extended; all the others are folded. And the elbow joint, hopelessly out of order, keeps balancing to and fro. The reader would do well to remember that the action takes place in Italy, where gestures are part of the language. And this is clearly an obscene, phallic gesture. The revolutionists, about to force the doors, would not mistake the gesture that "gives them the finger." They would think that they are being deliberately provoked. A blood bath is certain. As a last resort, the besieged bring hammers and, just as the attackers irrupt into the room, they are desperately trying to destroy the baleful prosthesis. The revolutionists encounter a man with a grotesquely contorted arm. It is an arm with almost spiral twists, a corkscrew-limb, an impossible upper extremity. What an extraordinary gesture!

Campanile's treatment of the subject of upper-limb expressiveness now reaches comical levels that belong in the absurd or surrealist domain. The frenzied revolutionists are suddenly frozen in puzzlement. What they see is not the Fascist salute, but not the Communist salute, either. It is an altogether new gesture of communication, an unprecedented and original salutation. "It is marvelous!" exclaims one of the rebels. And another one echoes: "It must be the embodiment of a new ideology!" The fact that no one knows the saluter is no impediment to his identification as a new, great leader. Is it not the normal course of revolutions to flow without restraint until a new leader emerges where no one expected him? Thus, the never-before beheld salute identifies the saluter as a man of destiny. And amidst cries of "Long live our leader!" the man with the artificial arm is carried off on the shoulders of the enthusiastic rebels.

Eventually, the new dictator imposes on the citizens of his troubled country the obligation to learn his charismatic salute. Prolonged training in special schools is required to learn it, and no one succeeds in mastering it. Only the great leader ever displays the salute in its perfect form. This is the source of his power over the masses, who idolize him on account of this marvelous ability. And, as other powerful men before him, the dictator with the amazing bendable arm becomes a despot. His repression is especially harsh against those who use the excuse of rheumatism and joint pain to avoid learning the new salute. His arbitrary measures will lead to his downfall. But the new revolution is not going to be easy, for the dictator is not without supporters. He counts among his most trusted followers orthopedic surgeons and physiotherapists: they became millionaires treating the sprains and subluxations of those who most eagerly tried to learn to master the dictatorship's obligatory salute.

MAESTOSO, RALLENTANDO

To break the body's free rhythms, or to alter its broad symmetries, does not always lead to the jocular results so craftily drawn by Campanile. An interruption in its sweeping equilibrium may take us to tragedy, as in bodily illnesses and gross deformities, or to ambiguity, or to mystery. Painters, and in particular por-

traitists of genius, have been aware of the remarkable poten-
tialities opened by alteration of the body's symmetry. The work
of Velázquez offers two remarkable examples of this expressive
dissymmetry: the portrait of Menippus, and those of the Count-
Duke of Olivares.[2]

Well known is the way by which the expressive potential is
unlocked. If by means of a piece of cardboard, or simply the
extended hand placed in front of our visual field, we obstruct
the view of one half of the portrayed face, we detect a certain
expression. If now we repeat the procedure to examine the
opposite half, we realize that the expression is a different one.
In his *Menippus,* Velázquez used this technique, probably without conscious intention, for the first time. One eyebrow is lifted
up, the other one lowered; one eye looks at us in placid contemplation, the other one glitters with an air of mordacity. And
without Velázquez departing one iota from that implacable
realism that made him paint a group of drunkards in a tavern,
or *bodegón,* to represent the triumph of Bacchus (where others
would have painted ethereal deities of Olympian mythology, as
required by convention), Velázquez delivers to us the substance
of Menippus. *This* man. The eccentric philosopher and farceur.
The satirical thinker of Gadara (now in Turkey), born to slaves,
who became immensely rich by begging and then through
usury. Complete with his only real and unique features.

The portrait of the Count-Duke of Olivares is another masterful exercise at revealing the duplicity of a mind through the
asymmetry of a face. But the complexity of the sitter's personality required all the mastery of a Velázquez, the "limner of
souls," to do it justice.

Don Gaspar de Guzmán, Count of Olivares (later made Duke
of San Lúcar, hence the double title) was, without question, as
ruthless an opportunist as they come.[3] The reader may know
him best as that mustachioed gentleman whom Velázquez immortalized in a famous equestrian portrait. Astride a spirited
steed that raises its front legs; all flowing sash and burnished
plate of armor; baton in hand, as in a gesture of guidance and

command; riding into a diaphanous horizon. With a name like Don Gaspar de Guzman y Pimentel, Ribera Velasco y de Tovar (all appellations refer to one man!), one is tempted to take him for the very image of seventeenth-century Spanish pomp, baroque and overwrought, a little like the incurved gentleman's mustache. A melancholy disappointment: this imposing general exhorting us to follow his brave example fought in no battle whatsoever. And this great statesman rose to power mainly on his ability to procure venal women for a corrupt and weak king. In effect, Philip IV gave himself to constant vainglorious activities, state ceremonies, festivals and religious processions, while Olivares appropriated for himself, with unhesitating calculation, the reins of power.

It is really not surprising that Olivares should have acceded to power through the back door. This was, apparently, the common way of access in his time. The temper of the people on the Iberian peninsula was one that saw no connection between a patient collective effort and the common weal. Fortunes were to be won or lost in one day. The fates of individuals, or of nations, were firmly believed to be at the mercy of unintelligible forces that passed all comprehension, and were neither foreseeable nor controllable. Adventurers and misfits, incapable of holding a decent job, were elevated to the highest honors, daily made lords of enormous provinces in the New World. The era of discoveries and colonization had bred a type of man eminently unsuited to sustain the progress of the country in those difficult times: fit for paroxysmal efforts, or heroic deeds, but incapable of the quiet tenacity that alone could save the country under the prevailing circumstances. Imagine a country of friars, lackeys, beggars, soldiers, serfs, and aristocrats. Imagine the best and most vital of its sons holding the gambler's mentality of win-all, lose-all, but disdaining as petty and meanhearted the quiet and patient effort necessary to set their house in order. Imagine this people convinced that God was on their side, since He had given them half the planet, and had once even deputized Saint James to lead the charges in their battles.

Imagine all this, and you will have a fair idea of the Spain of those times. And over this fundamentally chaotic people, this gigantic court of miracles, Olivares was supposed to rule.

This intolerant, egoistical, power-hungry man appoints Diego Velázquez as *pintor de Cámara* and sits patiently in front of him, exchanging casual comments to beguile hours of tedium. The result is several superb portraits. In one, he is the deceiving mounted general we all know. In another, he is an older gentleman clad in austere black cape, black doublet, and black stockings. He holds in his right hand a riding stick, because he has just come back from instructing the heir to the crown in the noble art of horsemanship, having decided to drop in, unannounced, into his talented protégé's shop. The latter (who did not consider himself a painter!) takes up his brushes and, without the benefit of a preliminary drawing or sketch—as was his custom—paints a masterful portrait in definitive, unhesitating, and powerful brushstrokes. In still another portrait (now part of the collection of the Duke of Westminster), the Count-Duke is at work in his capacity as tutor in the noble art of horsemanship. The Infante Baltazar Carlos has made some progress, and the Count-Duke basks in contentment at the learning ability of his pupil.

But the contented tutor has reasons to worry. Not the least of these is that the people see him as their enemy. There are disquieting rumors. They are saying that the ills of the country are largely due to him, which is only partly true. They say that the loss of important posts in Flanders and in France is due to his misrule, which is only partly false. And there is a rumor, colored by morbid and truculent nuance, which gives us a close-up view of the temper and mentality of the Spanish populace in those troubled times. They say that the king's lust drove him to slip into a convent, spurred by his sexual desire for a nun, Sister Margaret of the Cross. That the sister superior, trying to thwart the sacrilegious attempt, placed the intended victim on a bier, surrounded by burning candles and lilies, with a crucifix between her crossed arms, as if dead. That this theatrical ruse succeeded in saving Sister Margaret of the Cross from the unholy royal designs, but was not sufficient to dampen the royal satyriasis. That, thus frustrated in his original aim, the king turned his lust against the sister superior, who, in the end, submitted to the monarch's reprehensible desires. And here the popular imagination added finishing touches of an alarming nature, plainly showing that the most staunchly Catholic people on earth were also the most apt to imagine the absolute sacrilege, the supreme and most elaborate blasphemy. They say that the sister superior attired herself in white and blue, with the mantle of Our Lady of Conception. That she then copulated with the king at the foot of the main altar. And that all the while the monarch's accomplices, the Protonotary Don Juan de Villanueva and the Count-Duke of Olivares, stood on each side of the improvised bed, dangling censers suspended from silver chains, from which exhaled the fragrant smoke of incense.

A strong background in psychology is hardly necessary to interpret the origin of such popular rumors. They were, no doubt, the sickly offspring of strong minds uniquely gifted for color, realism, and ornamentation, yet driven to madness by extremes of want, disaffection, and misrule. On a different plane, the Spanish mind also sublimated this appalling alienation in the most exalted expressions of universal art. Contemporary with these gruesome tales, Cervantes wrote his works, and Velázquez recreated the light of nature.

At last the Count-Duke comes to sit again for the master. He is now older. He still wears black, austere Spanish gentleman that he is. All his clothing is still black, except the *gola* around his neck. He has met disillusion, fought intrigue, and daily tries his best to overcome anxiety. He does not know it yet, but his downfall is imminent. Why, he has even been shot at. It happened during a ceremonial salvo, in Aragón, when a discontented soldier fired at him. No matter. He trusts the Providence that saved him: the musket ball intended for his heart hit a dwarf, El Primo, who sat by his side. This, of course, could only mean that God still reserved him for other tasks, or so he wishes to believe. And so, once more, he sits for Velázquez, who takes up his brushes, and without benefit of preliminary sketch proceeds to pin his sitter's soul to the canvas, for all days to come.

We can see him today, at the Hermitage Museum, in Leningrad, just as he was when he sat that day, in Madrid, at the shop of his friend Diego Velázquez, *pintor de Cámara.* Middle-aged, jowls sagging, and upper lip sinking for lack of teeth, albeit somewhat dissimulated by a droopy mustache. Our first impression is perhaps to say, despite all the black in his clothing, "Here is a jolly old Spaniard of yore!" But if we look attentively, we discover behind the honeyed smile a certain trace of hypocrisy. Is it the little beady eyes, or the massive jaw, that give away the hidden craftiness? We cannot tell. But we know for certain that Velázquez has succeeded once more. He did not give us an idealized conception of hypocrisy. With all the force of Spanish realism he delivered to us *this* hypocrite. And if now we resort to the old trick of looking at one half of the face, then the other half, we are thrilled at the spectacle of Velázquez's superb craftsmanship. The left eye is inviting, open, frank and sincere: the eye of a jolly, olive-skinned Spaniard of yore. The right eye, however, sends a chill down our spine. It is the semi-hidden eye of a scheming, deceitful courtier. It is a cunning eye, sending forth emanations of malice, and waiting for us, as if to ambush us, behind the nasal bridge. We know that we are face to face with a man ready to stab us in the back, if he ever concludes that this action is to his profit; ready to stab his own mother, if by so doing he could reward, no matter how little, his immense and never assuaged political ambition.

LACRIMOSO (MA NON TROPPO)

It astonishes no one that we should so perceive the barely outlined subtleties of expression in a face. After all, it is to the face that we entrust the expression of mood. With a glance we confess, and with a furrowed brow we expostulate. Anxiety and

expectation announce themselves in the wrinkles of the forehead. And greed, or desire, though willfully concealed, betray
themselves in the trembling of a lip, or the distension of the
nares; just so, in the ancient tapestries, a cloven hoof or a
pointed tail sticking out from under Eden's foliage announced
that all was not well for the future of man. In Islam, to cover
the face of woman has been deemed necessary; some say for the
sake of modesty, some for the affirmation of women's subservi-
ence. But it may be that male hedonism in those lands invented
this unique pleasure: the solemnity, and the feeling of risk mingled with the trusting surrender of a woman who unveils her
face for her husband. At last, the moment comes for the singular
value of the face to be uncovered. And then the hieratic mystery of this screen for emission and reception of the radiations
of emotion is, suddenly, felt in all its power.

Yet it is not only the face that possesses this power of expression. An isolated part of the body can, like an ancient rhapsode,
spin tales for our entranced attention. In a short story by Luigi
Pirandello, "The Hand of the Poor Patient," it is a hand that
traces for us the relation of its vicissitudes.[4]

The narrator is a patient confined to a hospital ward for the
indigent. I do not suppose that too many people in the industrialized world would be able to picture what Pirandello means by
"a hospital ward for the indigent." Modern American hospitals,
housed in functionally designed buildings, run like efficient corporations, scrubbed cleaner than my dining room table on an
average day and replete with gleaming electronic equipment,
can give no idea of what Pirandello was trying to describe.
Nevertheless, the reality of his description is familiar to me, for
I spent a part of my life in precisely the setting depicted. And
in deference to my authority as ocular witness, I will allow
myself the short digression that is called for to recreate that
environment.

The building is gloomy, and ancient. It could have been a
lordly mansion in past, long-forgotten eras. It could have been
a public building that came to be placed under the protection

of the Ministry charged with the preservation of historical monuments. It might even have been a hospital from its inception, but now so ancient, so obsolete, that only major remodeling could bring it into consonance with the technical and architectural requirements of contemporary hospital medicine. Such remodeling is, of course, out of the question. The library is in a little-frequented, remote part of the building. It has dusty old volumes, many in noble leather bindings, and very few of any relevance to current medical practice. But this troubles no one, since physicians hardly use them, preferring to maintain their individual, meager supply of professional books and periodicals. Many are the details of ancient artistic beauty: a cupboard of sculpted wood in the kitchen, for which antiquarians would give a fortune; spouts shaped like gargoyles looming on outside walls; oriels with ornamented stone brackets; a central courtyard with a fountain decorated with colored tiles; and, at the entrance of a vaulted passage, surmounting the extrados of a graceful arch, a niche containing a statue of The Madonna and Child.

If you are a casual visitor, you cannot help but detect the noble charm exhaled from the hoary, venerable building. If you are a patient, the exhalation has for you less of the charm of the old, and more of the smell of the rancid. For, if you are a patient, you live in long, barracks-style halls, together with twenty or twenty-five other patients, who sleep in beds separated from each other by sliding curtains made of cloth, or by flimsy screens. Throughout the night you hear the moaning, the gurgling sound of stertorous respirations, the conversations of the ever-present relatives of other patients, the shouted orders of slovenly, ill-trained nurses, and the loud protestations of equally slatternly aides. And then, early in the morning, a group of medical students surround your bed. A grave professor lectures to them while holding your torso between his hands, and making you turn this way or that. You always do as he says: this is part of the natural order of things. Shortly thereafter, they all queue up to listen to your chest, to inspect your throat by making you gag, and to tap your abdomen with their cold fingers. If you are not stupid, you soon catch on. You provide the answers that they want to hear, and offer your body with sheepish submission to their manipulations. It is not all bad: in the long run this can be entertaining, and you are ready to go to extremes in order to break the drab monotony of the place. Slowly, the daily routines begin again. The veterans of the ward —indigents escaping a harsher fate outside the hospital—run errands for the nursing staff. Doctors come to extract yet more water from the abdomen of the patient on bed number twenty-five, or from the chest of number seventeen (the abbreviated denotation is not uncommon: your surname might easily turn into an Arabic number, albeit one pronounced with greater sympathy and warmth than was ever annexed to your family name). Often, usually in the afternoon or late in the evening, a commotion takes place when somebody dies, not far from your bedside. And for the rest of the day, after the body is taken away covered by bedsheets to the morgue, for the autopsy, a peculiar odor, half-phenol half-decomposition, pervades the long, rectangular room.

I am not describing a scene of a Dickensian novel. These are the conditions that I witnessed, some twenty-five years ago, in a Western country. It is not far-fetched to suppose that these conditions persist today, in many parts of the world. It is here that Pirandello places the patient of his story.

In this patient's ward, movable screens are not the fashion. Tents of white fabric separate one bed from the next. To his right side, a rent in the fabric allows him to peek into the neighboring patient's cubicle. All he can see is his neighbor's hand, as he removes it from under the bedsheets and abandons it on top of the covers. Yet this hand tells a complete story with its spontaneous movements. And the rhythm of the narrative is imprinted with the noble turns of the hand's unique language: lying langorously on its palm, or turning slowly on its dorsum; making a fist; grasping the sheets in a kind of crispatory movement; relaxing itself after a paroxysm.

It was the hand of a poor man "because, although washed with the thoroughness that is demanded by hospital regulations, there remained, in its yellowish leanness, a certain undetergeable dirt; which in the poor is not dirt properly speaking, but rather the patina of misery that no water can cleanse." Then, the patient observing through the rent in the fabric ponders what could be the trade of the observed hand, apparently too delicate for rude manual labor. From the position of the fingers, from the repeated gesture that they seem to adopt, and the callosities it developed, the hand avows its trade: it is the hand of a tailor. Often the thumb submits to the pressure of the index finger, as if the digits missed the reality to which they had been accustomed. And as if it persisted in the gestures for which it had been trained, the hand repeats the motions of grasping the tailor's scissors and steadying the fabrics to be cut.

From time to time the hand leaves the safety of the enclosure under the bedsheets and appears to direct itself toward the knee. Yet the knee, seen through the rent in the screen, is not touched by the hand. The hand seems to make a motion as if to caress the knee, but extends beyond it. What can this motion signify? Perhaps it extends to the head of a child, that reaches only to the level of the patient's knee. Perhaps the hand's gesture is the gesture that caresses the silky hair of a small child, a child that reaches only as high as that knee. Thus the hand says that it belongs to a tailor who is also a father.

On a certain morning, outside of visiting hours, a group of visitors surround the man with the communicative hand. Is he dying? Not likely, since the visitors are heard talking festively. But they do so in a low voice, in order not to disturb the other patients. It is also possible to discern that there is a priest in the group, and that a mirthful agitation is going on inside the crowded cubicle. At last the visitors leave. Now the view through the rent in the fabric is again clear. It is possible to see the hand that rests on the bedcovers. And this hand is changed: it wears a ring around the annular finger. A wedding! This was, no doubt, the reason for the commotion. They came to wed the poor patient. The poor patient and the poor hand! Weddings are not the same inside and outside the hospital. Outside, they are auspicious ceremonies open to the brightness of a future. Inside, they carry a different symbolism. They are ominous occurrences, forebodings of ill, precautions taken in anticipation of death.

Therefore the hand has made one more confession: it has said that the illness is incurable. And now it develops the saddening theme with its unique language. It says it with slow, fatigued motions; with gestures that seem purposeless; with long pauses, or interruptions of tiredness, and languor, and distraction.

I picture the hand of Pirandello's story as the servant of a mind that languishes and withers. Why fire orders at such a hand? To what purpose this waste of energy and direction? I imagine that if we could trade places with the mind that directs that hand, the world would look so different! And the hand itself would look different: a lean hand, emaciated and pale, incongruously ornamented with a shiny wedding band, set with gems. The ring, too wide for the finger, rotates loosely around the bony phalanxes and the wrinkled skin. Therefore, I imagine the mind at the controlling end of that hand pondering the meaning of the incongruence. And I picture the hand realizing the devastating logical consequence. The ring was granted on a short-term loan. An ornament has been put on today that will be taken off tomorrow. The ring that now embellishes the moving finger will be pulled off soon. And then the hand, bare, unadorned, will rot amidst worms and clay.

Is this not true for all parts of our body? But our precarious contentment will not be dislodged from its natural ignorance and obstinacy. We do not know when, and go on assuming, for no reason, that it will not be soon.

PIANGEVOLE

That a hand would tell wondrous tales is not surprising. For the hand is to the body as the reason to the soul. Andreas Laurentius (André Dulaurens), scholar of the sixteenth century, wrote:

"The hand is an instrument, but as it is the first instrument so it is the framer, yea, and employer of all other instruments. For not being framed for any particular vse it was capable of all: so as it may be justly compared to the soule, which as the Philosopher saith is, though not yet in deed yet in power and ability all things."[5] And later: "[the hands] are the vicars or substitutes or suffraganes of the speech, the interpreters of the secret language of our silent conceits, signifying to all men in a few letters as it were, by hieroglyphicks, what the very thoughts of our hearts are. . . ." But the question that we now ask is, would an immobile and quiet bodily part be able to speak to us so eloquently? A hand without its muscles, or a face devoid of skin and contractile parts that so vividly succeed in impressing upon it the movements of emotion, would they still pour out as powerful a message? Indeed. The language of the body cannot be stilled. But the body has a language all its own, and unfolds an eloquence that uses no words. He who could understand this language would be the ruler of nature.

A skull, crossed bones, an empty carcass: even these silent remains seem to address us. On his way to Ch'u, the philosopher Chuang Tzu (*circa* 300 B.C.) comes across a human skull lying on the road. It is a despicable object, whatever its former state may have been. This conviction is marked by the impatient gesture of the philosopher, who strikes it off the road with his horsewhip, and by the tone of haughtiness with which he addresses the useless aggregate of bleached bones: "How did you come to be what you are? Did you reach this state as a consequence of having lived in disaccord with the natural order of things? Or is your condition the just issue of the executioner's ax falling on you in retribution for some shameful act? Or did you come to this after some crime that stained the reputation of your family? Or was it only cold and famine that brought you here? Or did you simply die of old age?"

The skull has no audible answer. Chuang Tzu picks up the skull, and late that night finds for it a practical use that never occurred to Western mystics, and anchorites contemplating a *memento mori:* he uses it for a pillow when he lies down to sleep. Whether this familiarity had something to do with the nature of the philosopher's dreams that followed, no one can say. The fact is that the skull appears to him in a dream, and says: "You talked to me like one of those wandering sophists that make their living uttering vain arguments and paradoxes. For everything the living say is to the dead an entangled web of nonsense. The sayings of the philosophers are not excepted. Would you really like to hear how death is?"

"Yes," said Chuang Tzu.

"In death you will see neither the powerful above you, nor the humble below you. Neither sovereigns, nor servants. In death there is no tension, no conflict; you do not find the assiduous decay and renewal of the four seasons. Only ease is the measure of time. The greatest joys of a reigning king could not surpass the agreeable pleasantness of death."

Chuang Tzu was skeptical. He used all his sagacity in formulating a rejoinder. "Suppose," said he, "I could talk to the gods that control human existence. Suppose I were to ask them to restore your flesh, your limbs, your skin, and your organs of sense. Suppose they would grant all this, and also agree to return to you your parents, wife, children, friends, and neighbors. Would you accept the restitution?"

The skull frowned, as skulls are wont to do, and answered: "Can you suppose that anyone would willingly leave the state of perfect pleasantness to return to the life of toil and struggle that one finds among men?"[6]

The message is one of reassurance. Contemplation of human remains, Chuang Tzu seems to be saying, is a soothing experience. Bleached bones are a valid guarantee for an end to our troubles. Whatever our tensions may be, they shall end; and however intense our pleasures may seem, they shall be still greater when emptied of life's caducity and conflict. In the West, the body's discourse is interpreted differently. The silent words acquire the meaning of a formal lesson for the edification of the living. A skeleton addresses us from the lectern, like a learned professor, but it is not certain that we always catch the precise meaning of the lecturing.

The Western faith in the limitless possibilities of reason soon led observers to assume that the key to correct living could be deducted from the study of our mortal remains. Democritus of Abdera was judged mad by his contemporaries for his compulsion to cut in pieces the bodies of dead beasts. This early anatomist had no dreams of constructing an edifice of theory to explain bodily functions. His sole concern was to find the "seat of passions." And it was the nobility of his pursuit that led Hippocrates to exonerate him in the eyes of his contemporaries, adjudging him to be not a madman, but one among the wisest of men. For it is the foremost preoccupation of the wise man to know himself in order to find means to temper the tumultuous inner disarray that troubles the tranquillity of his life, and to control the passions that vex him daily, tossing him piteously like flotsam amidst unopposable waves. Therefore, a long line of moralist-anatomists takes origin in this Western tradition that interprets the oracular dictum, *nosce te ipsum,* "Know thyself," as an injunction to carry out anatomical dissections. He who knows himself knows that he is dust and ashes, and is thus safeguarded from arrogance. Well into the eighteenth century, anatomists profit from every opportunity to point out that study of their discipline carries with it the possibility of reaping moral benefits. In their dedications, in the prefatory remarks to their works, and interjected in the text of their descriptive treatises, the interpretations handed down from antiquity are not forgotten. The preeminence of their field is such, they say, that it must be made an indispensable part of the curriculum of liberal studies. For even the most exalted of men would be prevented from losing sight of the limitations of the human condition by a forced contemplation of our frail and wondrous inner framework. It is not in vain that their favorite historical quotation is a command of Philip of Macedon to his slave. Having vanquished the Athenians in the battle of Chaeronea, he ordered that every morning, to wake him up, his slave should tell him: "Get up, king, and remember that you are a man!," a reminder presumably intended to preserve him from vanity and excessive arrogance.

The language of mortal remains, however, does not receive a uniform interpretation. Some claim that the bared bones utter a harangue in favor of a democratic political system. Since the make-up of all men is substantially the same, the creation of immoderate privileges, or the bestowing of excessive honors to classes of individuals, is an unnatural and foolish practice. In Lucian's *Dialogues of the Dead,* a dead Diogenes can tell the equally dead Mausolus, renowned for his beauty: "Why should your skull be accounted better than mine? Both of them are bald and bare, both of us show our teeth in the same way, and have lost our eyes, and have snub noses now." The handsomest man, once come to the netherworld, presents a physiognomy no different from that of other men, unless it is in brittleness. And the wealthiest man, protesting his superiority, becomes the laughingstock of his companions in Hades. This is the sentiment that anatomists echo long after the Renaissance: in death we are all on equal footing. And if any consciousness survives after death, the roles might even be reversed; for the humble have nothing to regret, whereas the exalted, while bewailing the loss of their perquisites, must turn into clammy and swollen corpses, just like the others. Clearly, there was an element of the subversive in the study of anatomy. No good could be expected of extremists led by radical skeletons that would not be silenced.

Luckily, the skeleton speaks in a coded language. Therefore, it was possible to decipher its speech in more than one way. And the stalwart defenders of the established order were prompt to provide a transcription more in keeping with the sensible demands of good government. The body is a microcosm of society; in it is observed an admirable correspondence of various parts, a mutual agreement of diverse and manifold offices. He who attentively observes the use, the fashion, situation, and workmanship of anatomical organs, will perceive an admirable hierarchy, foreordained by God. In the words of Laurentius (loc. cit.): "You shall finde the rational faculty in the highest place, namely in the brain, compassed on every side with a scull; the faculty of anger, in the heart; the faculty of lust or desire in the liver; and therefore we may gather these lower and inferior faculties must bee serviceable and obedient to the higher, as to the queene and prince of them all." Accordingly, one ought not to be unduly stirred by what seemed an egalitarian, inflammatory speech uttered by bodily parts. The body's expressions may sound revolutionary to the ill informed, but a deeper science makes certain that the message will continue to support the status quo: ". . . if both princes and peasants would weigh and consider the mutuall offices betweene the principal and the ignoble parts, princes might vnderstand how to rule, and peasants how to obey."

Today, this kind of argument sways no one. Direct moral inferences can no longer be derived from the study of gross anatomy. We are at a stage where the merely visible has lost its eloquence. Medicine was almost entirely built by looking at the body; and even perceptions derived from other senses—as Michel Foucault outlined in *The Birth of the Clinic*—could be thought of as secondary or subservient functions of the eye. Nevertheless, we have reached the threshold of an era when the body will be studied not as the ingenious system that it was in the etchings of Vesalius and the many generations of his followers, but as a particular form of matter. As a physicochemical entity, it will be probed by intangible techniques. And like all matter, the body will be regarded one day as a mere "collection or grouping of events" in the universe. But the spectacle of concrete, individual death, of an inanimate, lifeless human body, or of an isolated part, like the skull, will continue to speak to us. It is by looking that we receive the message: the language of the body addresses only our gaze. And whatever else it might say (for the body's meanings continue to be controversial), it presents to us that forceful statement understood by the painters of *vanitas* portraits: "As you see me, you shall be. I, too, was once mobile, perceptive, and warm. You, who now course through life, remember that I was once as you are, and that you shall be, inevitably, as you see me."

Notes

GENERATION: PAST, PRESENT, AND FUTURE

1. Salvador E. Luria, *Life: The Unfinished Experiment* (New York: Scribner's, 1976).
2. François Jacob, *La logique du vivant: Une histoire de l'hérédité* (Paris: Gallimard, 1970). This book was hailed by the late Michel Foucault as the finest history of biology ever written. Hyperbole aside, it is a magnificent survey of the development of concepts of genetics in biology, written by a scientist who earned the Nobel Prize for his work in this field. Other works consulted for the elaboration of this essay were: Erik Nordenskiöld, *The History of Biology: A Survey,* trans. Leonard Bucknall Eyre (New York: Tudor Publishing Co., 1935), and Charles Singer, *A History of Biology* (New York: Henry Schuman, 1950).
3. Fray Benito Jerónimo Feijóo y Montenegro, *Influjo de la imaginación materna respecto al feto,* in Biblioteca de autores españoles, vol. 56 (Madrid: M. Rivadeneyra, 1863), pp. 472–476.
4. Dr. Jacobus [pseud.], *The Ethnology of the Sixth Sense: Studies and Researches into Its Abuses, Perversions, Follies, Anomalies, and Crimes* (Paris: C. Carrington, 1899).
5. V. R. Greenfield, "Wrongful Birth: What Is the Damage?" *Journal of the American Medical Association* 248 (Aug. 27, 1982): 926–27.
6. J. Coplan, "Wrongful Life and Wrongful Birth: New Concepts for the Pediatrician, *Pediatrics,*" 75 (January 1985): 65–67.

7. Quentin H. Stanford, ed., *The World's Population: Problems of Growth* (New York: Oxford University Press, 1972).
8. Charles F. Westoff and Norman B. Ryder, *The Contraceptive Revolution* (Princeton, N.J.: Princeton University Press, 1977). This work details the findings of the National Fertility Study, and contains a conscientious discussion of the methodological limitations applicable to the gathering of the data, as well as implications for public policy.
9. Council on Environmental Quality, *The Global 2000 Report to the President*, vol. 1 (0274–484) (Washington, D.C.: Government Printing Office, 1980).
10. O. Steeno, A. Adimojela, and J. Steeno, "Separation of X- and Y-Bearing Human Spermatozoa with the Sephadex Gel-Filtration Method," *Andrologia* 7 (1975): 95–97.
11. Neil G. Bennett, ed., *Sex Selection of Children* (New York: Academic Press, 1983).
12. Tabitha M. Powledge, "Toward a Moral Policy for Sex Choice," in Neil G. Bennett, *Sex Selection of Children*, chap. 9, 201ff.
13. Women outlive men in every country where maternal mortality has been reduced. In 1975, the United States Bureau of the Census stated that there were, in this country, 5,001,000 more women than men. For individuals 55 to 64 years of age, 63 percent of unmarried females were widowed, whereas only 22 percent of unmarried males were widowed. See Lester Hoyt Croft, *Sexuality in Later Life: A Counseling Guide for Physicians* (London: John Wright, 1982).
14. For a discussion of the impracticality of mass application of sex-choice technology, see John C. Fletcher's essay, "Ethics and Public Policy," which appears as chapter 10 in Neil Bennett's *Sex Selection of Children*. For an eloquent address regarding the perils of research on sex control, see the "classical" article by A. Etzioni, "Sex Control, Science and Society," *Science* 161 (1968): 1107–12.
15. Günter Grass, "Headbirths: Or the Germans Are Dying Out," trans. Ralph Manheim (New York: Fawcett Crest Books, 1984).

ON AGING

1. Lester Hoyt Croft, *Sexuality in Later Life: A Counseling Guide for Physicians* (London: John Wright, 1982).
2. G. M. Martin, "Syndromes of Accelerated Aging," *Journal of the National Cancer Institute. Monograph* 60 (1982): 241–47. In addi-

tion to this article, which contains a general classification of the syndromes of accelerated aging, the interested reader may consult descriptions of individual diseases manifesting acceleration of the aging process in numerous medical publications. Some of these are: Cockayne's syndrome is described in *Journal of Pediatrics* 75 (1969): 881; Werner's syndrome, in *Diabetes* 28 (1979): 389; and the "archetypal" disease, progeria, in *Journal of Pediatrics* 80 (April 1972): 714.

3. Alex Comfort, *The Biology of Senescence*, 3d ed. (New York: Elsevier, 1979).

4. The chronology of medical efforts to retard old age is quoted from Gairdner B. Moment, "The Ponce de Leon Trail Today," *Bioscience*, October 1975, pp. 623–28. Before the modern era of medical science, the most notable book on this subject was *Makrobiotik: The Art of Prolonging Life*, by Christopher William Hufeland, 2d English translation (London: J. Bell, 1797), a book that was a bestseller in its time. Of more recent memory, and thus of easier availability for the interested reader, is the work of Bogomolets, who claimed to have developed a serum to rejuvenate the connective tissues. See A. Bogomolets, *The Prolongation of Life* (New York: Duell, Sloan & Pearce, 1946). However, the nature of the serum remained uncertain, and his experiments could not be reproduced.

5. The work of the Rumanian investigators found its way into the most creditable scientific journals on the American continent. Experiments using "Gerovital" in rats are described in A. Aslan, A. Vrabiescu, C. Domiliscu, L. Campeanu, et al., "Long-term Treatment with Procaine (Gerovital H_3) in Albino Rats," *Journal of Gerontology* 20 (1965): 1–8. I have been unable to find reports of well-controlled trials of this substance on human beings. This did not discourage many prominent people from willingly submitting to this treatment. Chris Chase mentions Nikita Khrushchev, John F. Kennedy, and Konrad Adenauer among the "injectees" of Gerovital in her humorous and enjoyable book *The Great American Waistline: Putting It On and Taking It Off* (New York: Coward, McCann & Geoghegan, 1981).

SEXUAL UNDIFFERENTIATION

1. The life stories of Marguerite Malaure and Jean-Baptiste Grandjean had considerable notoriety, and are therefore discussed by most medical historians who deal with diseases characterized by ambig-

uous genitalia, or hermaphroditism. In the short biographical sketches presented here, I have followed mainly the article by Maurice Garçon, "Les tribulations des hermaphrodites," in *Histoire de la médecine (Paris);* vol. 12, no. 2 (February–March 1962), pages unnumbered.

2. Anatomical and medical aspects of hermaphroditism are well discussed in the textbook by Howard W. Jones and William Wallace Scott, *Hermaphroditism, Genital Anomalies, and Related Endocrine Disorders,* 2d ed. (Baltimore: Williams & Wilkins, 1971). Although medical treatises, as is well known, become obsolete a few years after publication, this impermanence relates mainly to diagnostic techniques and therapeutic methods; descriptions of gross anatomy generally remain unchanged. The reader interested in the developmental anatomy of these disorders may also consult the series of medical monographs *Birth Defects,* edited by Daniel Bergsma and published for the National Foundation–March of Dimes by Williams and Wilkins, Baltimore. In particular, vol. 7, no. 6, part X: *The Endocrine System* (May 1971).

3. The practices of this strange sect are quoted from Alain Daniélou, *Les quatre sens de la vie à l'Inde traditionelle* (Paris: Librairie Académique, 1963). Mention should also be made, in this context, of the Tantric practices of India. The mystical-spiritual cult of Tantra has as one of its aims to make people consciously aware that human beings are composed of intermixed elements from both sexes. However, the tenets of this belief seem to be directed mostly at men. Tantra has been characterized, therefore, as "a quest for androgyny." Followers do not try to deny their maleness, but strive to realize all the feminine aspects of the self. They claim that psychic bisexuality is not only desirable, but possible through a series of physical and mental exercises connected with the sexual act. An interesting discussion of Tantra by an Indian psychiatrist trained in the West may be found in the book by Sudhir Kakar, *Shamans, Mystics and Doctors: A Psychological Inquiry into India and Its Healing Traditions* (New York: Knopf, 1982), pp. 151–90.

4. Luis Buñel: *Mi último suspiro* (Barcelona: Plaza & Janes, 1982). Translated from the French (*Mon dernier soupir* [Paris: Editions Robert Laffont, 1982]) by Ana Maria de la Fuente.

5. My source for women acting as male impersonators was E. J. Dingwall; *Some Human Oddities* (London: Home & Van Thal, 1947). I know of no readily available biography of "Count Balmori," and I have but sketched some personal reminiscences of the noted scandals.

6. Female impersonation by male actors and entertainers in Japan is well described in chapter 7, entitled "The Third Sex," of Ian Buruma's recent book, *Behind the Mask* (New York: Meridian Books, 1984). I acknowledge my debt to this perceptive study for some of the anecdotes of Japanese show business.

MORS REPENTINA: AN ESSAY ON THREE FORMS OF SUDDEN DEATH

1. According to Isaac Disraeli's *Curiosities in Literature,* 14th ed., vol. 2 (New York: W. J. Widdleton, 1875), the verses composed by Marguerite of Austria for her own epitaph, while under the emotional impact of the raging storm, were these. The translation is Disraeli's.

> *Cy gist Margot, la gente demoiselle*
> *Qu'eut deux maris et si mourut pucelle.*

> Beneath this tomb is gentle Margot laid
> Who had two husbands, yet died a maid.

Judging by this sample, the emotional tension provoked by a storm does little to enhance poetic inspiration. We agree with Disraeli: she should have said her prayers. In contrast, the poem composed by André Chénier while waiting for his turn to be guillotined has a moving romantic pathos, suggesting that the proximity of death may be capable of stirring talent to exertion, provided, however, that talent there be. Apparently Chénier had set out to compose a sonnet, the one that starts with the line: *"Comme un dernier rayon, comme un dernier zéphyre . . ."* (Like a last ray, like a last zephyr . . .). He had proceeded to the ninth line: *"Le sommeil du tombeau pressera ma paupière—"* (The sleep of the grave will weigh upon my brow—), when his task was interrupted by the arrival of the executioner, who dragged him to the guillotine. The sonnet was left unfinished.

2. In one version, death by lightning was also the fate that befell Romulus. In a less poetic version, he was murdered by Roman senators. Much political agitation followed his disappearance, but Proculeius faced an irritated mob, and was able to deflect its wrath by saying in a speech that Romulus had appeared to him and assured him that the future of the country was safe under his protection, for he had now become a god (Livy I, 16). This "miracle" calmed the people, and sent them to build altars to the deified

politician. Later, Diderot used this historical episode to ridicule miracles, apparitions, and fake supernatural occurrences (*Pensées Philosophiques* 49). The freethinker does not fear hurting his contemporaries' religious susceptibilities; in retelling the episode, Diderot makes Proculeius say that Romulus has gone to heaven, where he "sits to the right of Jupiter," in an obvious parallel to Christ.

3. R. K. Haugen, "The Café Coronary: Sudden Deaths in Restaurants," *Journal of the American Medical Association* 186 (Oct. 12, 1963): 142–43.

4. Quoted in H. J. Heimlich and M. H. Uhley, "Historical Review of the Literature on Choking," *Ciba Clinical Symposia* 31 (1979): 24–32.

5. R. E. Mittelman and C. V. Wetli, "The Fatal Café Coronary: Foreign-Body Airway Obstruction," *Journal of the American Medical Association* 247 (Mar. 5, 1982): 1285–88.

6. C. S. Harris, S. P. Baker, G. A. Smith, and R. M. Harris, "Childhood Asphyxiation by Food: A National Analysis and Overview," *Journal of the American Medical Association* 251 (May 4, 1984): 2231–35.

7. This definition of asphyxia appeared in the *Lexicon Medicum Graeco-Latinum,* by Steven Blankaart (1650–1702), first published in Amsterdam in 1679. The Latin edition (Jena: Muller, 1683) was published in facsimile by Olms of Hildesheim in 1973. Today a curiosity of the history of medicine, Blankaart's dictionary remained for many years an important medical reference text. More than twenty editions were printed, and it was often quoted until well into the eighteenth century.

8. For a review of the medical aspects of the various diseases characterized by attacks of apnea, see Christian Guilleminault, Ara Tilkian and William C. Dement, "The Sleep Apnea Syndromes," *Annual Review of Medicine* 27 (1976): 465–84.

9. Among the numerous works devoted to Fuseli, I would like to call attention to a fine critical study of what has become perhaps his best known painting: Nicolas Powell, *Fuseli: The Nightmare* (New York: The Viking Press, 1972).

10. Gregory of Nyssa's essay, "On Infants' Early Deaths," is available in English translation in *Select Writings and Letters of Gregory, Bishop of Nyssa,* trans. William Moore and Henry Austin Wilson. (New York: The Christian Literature Co., 1893), pp. 372–81.

OUR PREDACEOUS NATURE

1. The most comprehensive treatise on the utilization of insects as food remains, to this date, the work entitled *Insects as Human Food: A Chapter in the Ecology of Man,* by Friedrich S. Bodenheimer (The Hague: W. Junk, 1951).

2. Marston Bates, *Gluttons and Libertines: Human Problems of Being Natural* (New York: Random House, 1967).

3. The most prevalent alimentary prejudices and their geographic distribution are discussed by Frederick J. Simoons in his book *Eat Not This Flesh: Food Avoidances in the Old World* (Madison, Wis.: University of Wisconsin Press, 1961).

4. To the now internationally famous cardiovascular surgeon Dr. Michael DeBakey is owed the most comprehensive medical article on bezoars, which he wrote in collaboration with Dr. Alton Ochsner (M. De Bakey and A. Ochsner, "Bezoars and Concretions," *Surgery* 4 [December 1938]: 934–63, and [January 1939]): 132–69—almost fifty years ago. Allowing for advances in diagnostic techniques that have become available since the communication by DeBakey and Ochsner, this two-part article remains an authoritative study on the origin of bezoars, their associated clinical manifestations, and their appropriate surgical treatment. It is also a rich source of bibliography on historical aspects of these strange objects (342 references). I also consulted the following sources: R. Matas, "Hair Balls, or Hair Casts of the Stomach and Gastrointestinal Tract: With Special Reference to Their Pre-operative Diagnosis by Radiographic Methods of Investigation, and a Report of a Large Hair Cast of the Stomach Successfully Removed by Gastrostomy," *Surgery, Gynecology and Obstetrics* 21 (1915): 594–608. and Edwin D. Vaughn, John L. Sawyers and William H. Scott, "The Rapunzel Syndrome: An Unusual Complication of Intestinal Bezoar," *Surgery* 63 (February 1968): 339–43.

To the strange ideas on the origin of bezoars discussed in this section may be added another one, yet more fantastic, if such were possible. Throughout antiquity and the Middle Ages, it was widely believed that bezoars could originate from the solidified tears of deer, or of horses. The Arab physician Avenzoar, who lived in Spain in the eleventh century, maintained that certain deer, when bitten by venomous serpents, swam into rivers and remained submerged until they felt the effect of the venom to subside. At this point they shed a large tear that solidified upon the deer leaving the water. Scribonius Largus, Roman physician of the first century A.D., and author of one of the first works on pharmacology, *De compositione medicamentorum*, also subscribed to the belief that bezoars originate from the inner canthus of the eyes of deer, from solidification of tears, and added the quaint detail that Sicilian hunters gathered them eagerly. There is a brief mention of these superstitions in the work of the sixteenth-century scholar and physician Laurent Joubert, *Treatise on Laughter*, recently translated by Gregory David de Rocher (Tuscaloosa, Ala.: University of Alabama Press, 1980), p. 99.

5. An excellent and concise review of past theories on gastric physiology, to which I owe the historical information and the Hunterian quotation here presented, is that of William C. Rose. It appears in the preface to a reimpression of the doctoral thesis of John R. Young, a little-known American pioneer of the modern era of investigation of the biochemistry of gastric digestion. See John R. Young, *An Experimental Inquiry into the Principles of Nutrition and the Digestive Process* (1803, reprint, Urbana-Champaign, Ill.: The Board of Trustees of the University of Illinois, 1959).

6. The belief that the stomach works like a stove is traced by anthropologists Farb and Armelagos to persistence of old ideas derived from humoral medicine. Precautionary measures having little scientific foundation, such as avoidance of bathing after eating, or aversion to drinking cold water with meals, are linked to the belief that an elevation of bodily temperature, mainly inside the stomach, contributes to the digestive process. In the opinion of Farb and Armelagos, the saying "Feed a cold, starve a fever" is an example of the persistence of the notion that hot-cold principles control bodily functions. A heavy meal, by generating higher temperatures, would remedy a cold; fasting, presumably reducing temperature, would tend to counteract a fever. See Peter Farb and George Armelagos, *Consuming Passions: The Anthropology of Eating* (Boston: Houghton Mifflin, 1980).

7. After this part of the present essay had been published in a magazine (*The Sciences,* bimonthly publication of the New York Academy of Sciences, November–December 1985, pp. 18–25), under the title "The Rapunzel Syndrome," I received a letter from Dr. Mark L. Taff, Deputy Medical Examiner of the County of Nassau, in the State of New York. In this letter was included a copy of a scientific communication written by Drs. Gabriel Yelin, Mark L. Taff, and George E. Sadowski that reported the autopsy findings in an individual who swallowed two hundred and seventy-five United States coins, and died from copper poisoning. The copper was absorbed from the partially corroded coins. Striking as this case

appears, it is not a record. The *Guinness Book of Records* describes the ingestion of 424 coins and 27 pieces of wire by a man fifty-four years old (London: Guinness Superlatives Ltd., 1972, p. 22). J. M. Dixon and collaborators have described the ingestion of keys, coins, and a teaspoon by a mentally disturbed woman forty-three years old. The keys and coins were eventually passed *per rectum*, but the spoon was retained. By serial X-ray studies performed over the ensuing fifteen months, it could be seen that the head of the spoon was slowly corroded and eventually dissolved. See J. M. Dixon, C. P. Armstrong, and G. C. Davies, "Corrosion of Swallowed Foreign Body," *Journal of the Royal Society of Medicine* 75 (1982): 567–68. I acknowledge my gratitude to Dr. Mark L. Taff for the privilege of bringing the scholarly communication that he co-authored to my attention, before its publication in the forensic medical literature, and for alerting me to the existence of previously reported instances of comparable nature. Not included in their review (as having been of no significant pathologic consequence) was the report "A Historic Foreign Body," by T. B. Layton, in the *British Medical Journal* of January 4, 1930, p. 24. Prince Friedrich Wilhelm I, son of Kurfurst Friedrich Wilhelm, Elector of Brandenburg, swallowed a small silver shoe buckle at the age of five years, on December 31, 1692. There was great commotion in the palace, and wild wailing of nurses, but, according to Thomas Carlyle's narrative in his biography of Frederick the Great, "a few grains of rhubarb returned it to the light of day." According to Layton, the silver buckle was still being exhibited at the Hohenzollern Museum at the Château of Monbijon, in Room 35, at the time of his report. By comparison with the spectacular ingestions described in the medical literature, this incident appears trivial. Nevertheless, the potential historical consequences were momentous, and the shoe buckle was duly catalogued and elevated to the status of a museum piece. "A very ordinary buckle," wrote the author of the medical report, "but had it not passed the larynx, no Frederick the Great might have been begotten, and the history of Europe would have changed."

8. The interesting statements made by the young South American survivors of the plane crash to an eager crowd of journalists can be read in the Reuter reports in *The Times* of London, of December 28 and 30, 1972, and *The New York Times* of January 1, 1973. At least one book was written based on this occurrence. It is entitled *Alive*, by Piers Paul Read (Philadelphia: Lippincott, 1974).

9. Many are the hair-raising accounts of the early explorers who first

came across cannibalistic practices in primitive societies. Works consulted were R. G. Berry, "The Sierra Leone Cannibals," *Proceedings of the Royal Irish Academy* 30 (1912): 419; Garry Hogg, *Cannibalism and Human Sacrifice* (New York: Citadel, 1966), pp. 29–30; Reay Tannahill, *Flesh and Blood: A History of the Cannibal Complex* (London: Hamish Hamilton, 1975); Ronald M. Berndt, *Excess and Restraint: Social Control Among a New Guinea Mountain People* (Chicago: University of Chicago Press, 1962).

10. Eli Sagan, *Cannibalism, Human Aggression and Cultural Form* (New York: Harper & Row, 1974).

11. Quoted by Frank Lestrignant in a scholarly article entitled "Rage, fureur, folie cannibales: Le Scythe et le Brésilien," published in *La Folie et le Corps,* studies gathered by Jean Céard with the collaboration of Pierre Naudin and Michel Simonin (Paris: Presses de l'École Normale Supérieure, 1985).

12. The "History of East Chou's Many States" is a Chinese classic attributed to the chronicler Yu Xiào-Yu. I gratefully acknowledge the help of my wife, Dr. Wei Hsueh, in translating this account, which appears in volume 22, chapter 85, of the Chinese text (Taipei: Wen Jèn Publishers, 1972).

13. The pertinence of the study of cannibalism today seems to be indicated by interest in this subject in fields as diverse as medical epidemiology and jurisprudence. Knowledge of the natural history of "slow viruses" benefited from study of the cannibalistic practices of tribesmen in New Guinea, who acquired virus-induced degenerative diseases of the central nervous system by eating the brains of infected human beings. Slow viruses affect people in developed societies, but the prototype of these illnesses is "Kuru," a disease of New Guinea aborigines. See Robert Glasse, "Cannibalism in the Kuru Region of New Guinea," *Transactions of the New York Academy of Sciences,* 2d series, 29 (1967): 748–54. Concerning the relationship of studies on cannibalism and law, a recently published book (W. A. Brian Simpson, *Cannibalism and the Common Law* [Chicago: University of Chicago Press, 1985]) attests to the continuing interest of jurisconsults and legal historians in this matter. The book deals with the legal precedents set by the 1884 death sentence passed by the Queen's Bench Division against two seamen who, pushed by their instinct of survival, murdered and ate a shipmate aboard the *Mignonette.* The important legal issue bears on the "defense of necessity" and weighs the need to survive against a moral code that respects the sanctity of life.

14. Bruno Bettelheim, *The Uses of Enchantment: The Meaning and Importance of Fairy Tales* (New York: Knopf, 1976).

THE FEMALE BREAST

1. *La Grande Encyclopédie,* vol. 22 (Paris: Societé Anonyme de la Grande Encyclopédie, n.d.). Let us note that the curious remarks on breast shape are repeated, obviously without the Gallic flair, in a German encyclopedia of recent publication. The Brockhaus Encyclopedia states, under the entry *Brustdrüsen: "Flach oder scheibenförmig sind sie haüfig bei Mongoloiden, Halbkugelform herrscht in Europe vor, Kegelform bei den Negrinnen"* (Der Grosse Brockhaus [Wiesbaden: F. A. Brockhaus, 1978], vol. 2, p. 331). I do not know what the current status is of this matter in the corpus of knowledge of physical anthropology. But it suffices for me to see it discussed by German encyclopedists to convince me that the subject is a ponderous one, well beyond the purview of girl-watchers posted on street corners.

2. Quoted in Daniel de Moulin, *A Short History of Breast Cancer* (Hinsham, MA: Martin Nijhoff, 1983. Distributed in the United States and Canada by Kluwer, Boston).

3. Bruno Roy, "L'humour érotique au XVe siecle," in *L'érotisme au Moyen Age,* chap. 8 (Montreal: Aurore, 1977).

4. Quotations on breast-related terms, euphemistic and unvarnished, ancient and modern, are all from the superb work of Peter Fryer, *Mrs. Grundy: Studies on English Prudery* (New York: House & Maxwell, 1964).

5. Quoted in Prudence Glynn, *Skin to Skin: Eroticism in Dress* (New York: Oxford University Press, 1982).

6. Gordon Rattray Taylor, *The Angel Makers* (London: Heinemann, 1958).

7. The saying is attributed to C. B. Goodhart, of Caius College, Cambridge, in Anthony Smith, *The Body* (New York: Walker and Co., 1965).

8. The introduction of whalebone for making rigid corsets is attributed to Ysabeau de Bavière (Maurice Leloir, *Dictionnaire du costume* [Paris: Librairie Gründ, 1951]), who was the subject of a not very flattering biography by none other than the Marquis de Sade. The history of the modern brassière is difficult to trace, because the name was given to different garments. Brassière, bra-

cière, or brasserole was a type of short, sleeveless camisole worn by little girls and women after childbirth since the Middle Ages. A short, quilted jacket worn by men from 1600 to 1670 was given the same name by Molière, presumably as a joke. There followed the empire of the high-boned corset, maleficient creation of the *empoisonneuse* Ysabeau de Bavière. A new Perseus, Paul Poiret is credited with the liberation of the imprisoned female bosom (see R. Turner Wilcox, *The Dictionary of Costume* [New York: Scribner's, 1969].) He came to the rescue with the creation of his Empire style in 1912, then rode into the setting sun after the new garment became established and endured well into the 1920s.

9. Saint Agatha figures in all Greek and Latin martyrologies. She is protectress of the Order of Malta. Pope Symmacus (498–515) ordered the construction of a basilica with a baptistery on the Via Aurelia, two miles from Rome, in honor of the saint. Having turned down the lewd propositions of Quintianus, who, in Baring-Gould's phrase, "admired her exceedingly," she was handed over to a wicked woman who kept a house of prostitution with her six daughters. The name of the infamous madam was, quite fittingly, Aphrodisia. (See S. Baring-Gould, *The Lives of the Saints* [Edinburgh: John Grant, 1914], vol. 2, p. 136.) "In this dreadful place," says Butler, "she suffered assaults and stratagems upon her honour, more terrible to her than death." But the saint stood firm, and she was tortured, suffering the amputation of her breasts (Alban Butler, *The Lives of the Saints*, revised and edited by Herbert Thurston [London: Burns, Oates and Washburne, 1926–38], vol. 2 (1930), pp. 80–81).

10. For the sketch of the life of Raymond Llull I have followed Marcelino Menéndez y Pelayo, *Historia de los españoles heterodoxos* (Buenos Aires: Espasa Calpe Argentina, 1951), vol. 3, pp. 231–38.

THE ANORECTUM

1. William S. Haubrich, "Anatomy of the Colon," in J. Edward Bark, ed., *Bockus Gastroenterology*, 4th ed. (Philadelphia: W. B. Saunders, 1985).

2. St. John Chrysostom, *Homilies on the Gospels of Saint Matthew*, trans. and ed. by Philip Schaf (New York: Scribner's, 1908).

3. Robertson Davies, *The Rebel Angels* (New York: Penguin Books, 1983).

4. Comments on the work of Francisco de Quevedo, as well as bio-

graphical notes, were based on the complete works published as *Obras completas: Prosa,* 6th ed. (Madrid: Aguilar, 1969). All translations are my own responsibility.

5. Octavio Paz, *Conjunctions and Disjunctions,* trans. Helen R. Lane (New York: Seaver Books, 1982).
6. Ian Gibson, *The English Vice: Beatings, Sex and Shame in Victorian England and After* (London: Duckworth, 1978).
7. Marcel Pagnol, *Notes sur le rire* (Paris: Editions Nagel, 1947).

THE BODY AND THE EMOTIONS

1. Juan Luis Vives, *Tratado del alma* (Buenos Aires: Espasa-Calpe Argentina, S.A., Colección Austral, 1942). In Vives's essay on laughter, published in this book, the Spanish scholar is merely repeating an ancient belief, already expressed by Aristotle in *De Partibus Animalum,* book 3, chap. 10, 673a. A note in the Oxford edition (English translation by William Ogle, under the editorship of J. A. Smith and W. D. Ross [London: Oxford University Press, 1958]) states that Aristotle had maintained that instant death usually follows diaphragmatic rupture, and that the face of the deceased invariably assumes the peculiar smiling expression known as *Risus Sardonicus.* These ideas were widely adopted throughout the Middle Ages and into the Renaissance. Laurent Joubert (1529–1582), Montpellier physician, discusses laughter accompanying an injured diaphragm in book 2, chap. 4, of his *Treatise on Laughter* (see note 15 below).
2. W. F. Fry and C. Rader, "The Respiratory Component of Mirthful Laughter," *Journal of Biological Psychology* 19 (1977): 39–50.
3. Norman Cousins, "Anatomy of an Illness" (as perceived by the patient), *New England Journal of Medicine* 295 (1976): 1459–63.
4. L. Lehtinen and A. Kivalo, "Laughter Epilepsy," *Acta Neurologica Scandinavica* 41 (1965): 255–61.
5. N. A. Leopold, "Gaze-Induced Laughter," *Journal of Neurology, Neurosurgery and Psychiatry* (London) 40 (1977): 815–17.
6. Quoted by Donald W. Black in his article "Pathological Laughter: A Review of the Literature," *Journal of Nervous and Mental Diseases* 170 (1982): 67–71.
7. Except when otherwise indicated by a corresponding note, the following work was the source of quotations of philosophers' comments on and definitions of the nature of the comic: Ralph Piddington, *The Psychology of Laughter: A Study in Social Adaptation,*

(London: Adelphi, 1933). This work may be used as ready reference by those interested in the different philosophical points of view on the subject of laughter and the comic.

8. Marcel Pagnol, *Notes sur le rire* (Paris: Editions Nagel, 1947).

9. This "imitation" of Seneca originated from my fond memory of the famous work of Lucius Anneus Seneca, *De Ira*, which I read in my youth in the superb Spanish translation of Lorenzo Riber published, as part of the complete works of the Roman philosopher, by Aguilar (*Obras Completas de Lucio Aneo Seneca* [Madrid: Aguilar S.A., 1949]). It convinced me that Seneca can have no imitators: any addition, deletion, or alteration is detrimental to his perfect work.

10. Alain was the pseudonym of Emile-Auguste Chartier (1868–1951), superb essayist, philosopher, and man of exemplary life. The extraordinary literary quality of his work taxes to the limit attempts at translation, which may be the reason for the relatively restricted diffusion of his work in America. I take responsibility for the quotations of his ideas on desire, published in *Les Passions et la Sagesse* (Paris: Gallimard, Bibliothèque de la Pléiade, 1960), chap. 15, *"Le désir,* pp. 386–88.

11. William R. Charlesworth and Mary Anne Kreutzer, "Facial Expressions of Infants and Children," in Paul Ekman, ed., *Darwin and Facial Expression: A Century of Research in Review* (New York: Academic Press, 1973), chap. 3, pp. 91–168.

12. Patrick D. Trevor-Roper, *The Eye and Its Disorders* (Oxford: Blackwell Scientific Publications, 1974), footnote p. 133.

13. R. B. Zajonc, "Emotion and Facial Efference: A Theory Reclaimed," *Science* 228 (April 1985): 15–21.

14. Plutarch's *Moralia,* trans. Philip H. DeLacy and Benedict Einarson (London: William Heinemann, 1959), vol. 7, p. 593.

15. Laurent Joubert, *Treatise on Laughter,* trans. Gregory David de Rocher (Tuscaloosa, Ala.: The University of Alabama Press, 1980).

THREE THEORISTS OF EMOTION

1. All quotations from the work of Descartes refer to the *Treatise on the Passions of the Soul.* Translations are my own responsibility, from *Les Passions de l'Âme,* in René Descartes, *Oeuvres et Lettres* (Paris: Gallimard, Bibliothèque de la Pléiade, 1953), pp. 691–802.

2. All quotations from William James (1842–1910) refer to his monograph "The Emotions." I used the version reprinted in *Psychology*

Classics, vol. 1, edited by Knight Dunlap (Baltimore: Williams & Wilkins Co., 1922).

3. Walter B. Cannon, *Bodily Changes in Pain, Hunger, Fear and Rage* (New York: Appleton-Century, 1927).

4. M. B. Arnold, ed., *The Nature of Emotion* (London: Penguin Books, 1968).

5. Jean Paul Sartre, *Esquisse d'une théorie des émotions,* in *Actualités Scientifiques et Industrielles,* no. 838 (Paris: Herman et Cie., 1939).

6. William Lyons, *Emotion* (New York: Cambridge University Press, 1980).

7. Søren Kierkegaard, "The Unhappiest Man," In *Either/Or,* vol. 1, trans. David F. Swenson and Lillian M. Swenson with revisions by Howard A. Johnson (Princeton, N.J.: Princeton University Press, 1971), pp. 215–28.

SOME EXPRESSIONS OF THE BODY (IN FOUR MOVEMENTS)

1. Achille Campanile, *L'eroe, o si direbbe che a uno squillo di tromba* . . . (Milan: Rizzoli, 1976).

2. For a learned appraisal of the work of Velázquez, in particular the several portraits of the Count-Duke of Olivares, see the study by Vladimir Kemenov, *Velázquez in Soviet Museums: Analysis and Interpretation of the Paintings in the Context of His Oeuvre* (Leningrad: Aurora Art Publishers, 1977).

3. The life and times of the Count-Duke of Olivares may be read in Gregorio Marañón, *El Conde-Duque de Olivares* (Madrid: Espasa-Calpe, S.A., 1965).

4. Luigi Pirandello, "La mano del malato povero," in *Novelle per un anno: Il viaggio,* 4th ed. (Milan: A. Mondadori, 1982).

5. Andreas Laurentius, *Mikrokosmographia: A Description of the Body of Man,* trans. from Latin by Helkiah Crooke (London, 1615), book 13, chap. 3, "De manuum prestantia."

6. *The Sayings of Chuang Tzu,* trans. James R. Ware (Taiwan: Confucius Publishing Co., n.d.).